COMPLETE EASY

ACID REFLUX

DIET PLAN

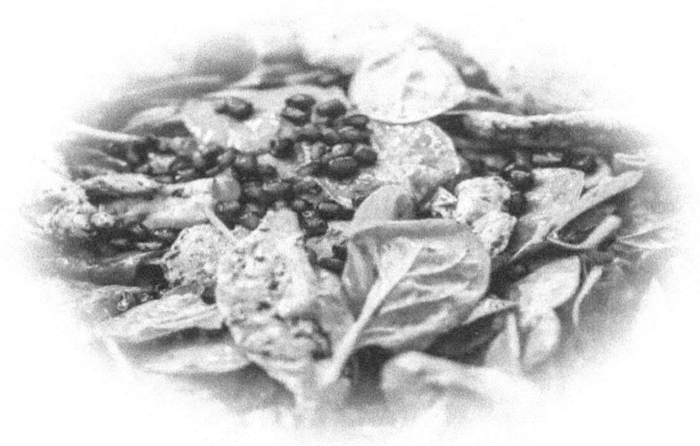

Escape Plan and Healthy Heartburn-friendly Recipes to Heal Your GERD & LPR

Dr. Olivier Michael

Copyright © 2024 by [Dr. Olivier Michael]

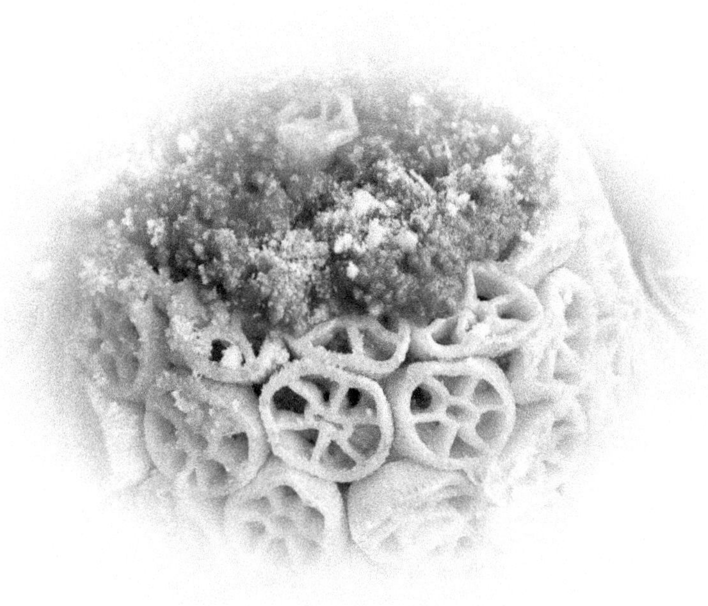

TABLE OF CONTENTS

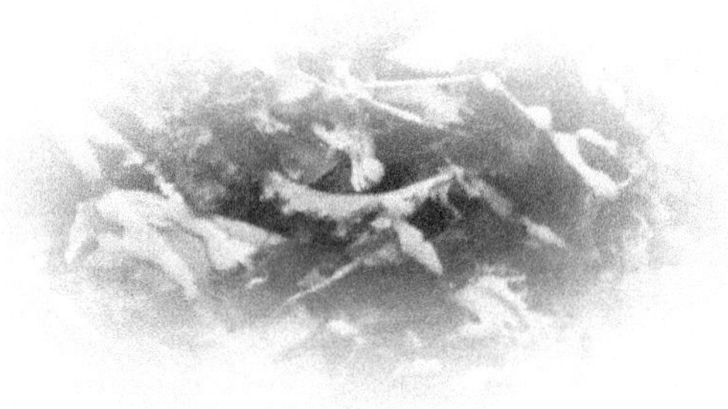

INTRODUCTION

There was a time when Tracy was caught in a vicious cycle of unease and annoyance. He fought the never-ending symptoms of both GERD (Gastroesophageal Reflux Disease) and LPR (Laryngopharyngeal Reflux) for years, never managing to find any respite from the burning feeling in his chest or the continuous irritation in his throat.

Tracy was desperate to find a way back to his former level of health and energy. Nothing appeared to provide long-lasting comfort despite the multiple drugs he took, fad diets he attempted, and counsel from various medical specialists. He had the impression that there was no way out and he was stuck in an endless labyrinth.

Tracy found solace in the "Complete Easy Acid Reflux Diet Plan" cookbook, nevertheless, just as he was about to give up. Tracy was intrigued by the idea of using nutritious meals as a natural healing method, so she excitedly turned to the pages, reading every word with a renewed feeling of hope.

With newfound information and resolve, Tracy decided to change the way he ate, embracing the appetizing and healthful dishes that were printed throughout the cookbook. Every meal, including the tasty quinoa-stuffed bell peppers and the cozy oatmeal with banana and nut butter, was specifically designed to calm his stomach and lessen his symptoms.

Tracy saw a startling shift in him as the days stretched into weeks and the weeks into months. He felt a wave of calm and comfort sweep over him for the first time in years as the searing feeling in his chest started to diminish and the irritation in his throat subsided.

Tracy's quest for recovery turned from a dream into a reality with every mouthful of healthful, acid-reflux-friendly food. Tracy beat the odds and permanently regained his health and energy thanks to the power of food and the advice of this "Complete Easy Acid Reflux Diet Plan" cookbook. Although he enjoyed the taste of freedom, he realized that his story—a monument to the healing potential of taking care of one's body as well as one's soul—was just getting started.

"Say goodbye to GERD"

REASONS FOR ACID REFLUX AT THE BASIS

The common digestive disorder known as acid reflux may be caused by several factors that have physiological and behavioral origins. The lower esophageal sphincter, a muscle that separates the stomach and esophagus, is a major contributor.

Weakened it is. Stomach acid may reflux into the esophagus when this muscle isn't performing correctly, producing discomfort and irritation. Furthermore, by creating more stomach acid or relaxing the LES, some dietary choices such as eating fatty meals, hot or acidic foods, coffee, and alcohol can make symptoms worse.

By increasing pressure on the abdomen or disturbing the natural balance of digestive processes, lifestyle factors like obesity, smoking, and certain drugs may further cause acid reflux. People are better prepared to manage and prevent acid reflux for improved digestive health when they are aware of these underlying factors.

UNDERSTOOD THE ACID REFLUX DIET

1. Identify Food Triggers: With your acid reflux, certain meals may make it worse. These frequently include chocolate, coffee, citrus fruits, tomatoes, chocolate-covered meals, fatty foods, and fizzy beverages. To reduce acid reflux, it's crucial you understand and stay away from particular trigger foods.

2. Take Advantage of Low-Acid Options: To minimize your probability of acid reflux flare-ups, eat low-acid foods. This means including more vegetables like broccoli, carrots, and green beans in your diet along with fruits like bananas, apples, and pears.

3. Keep an Eye on Portion Sizes: Overindulging in food puts greater pressure on your stomach, which may increase acid reflux symptoms. To minimize the probability of reflux episodes, check what you eat and keep clear of big meals, particularly soon before bed.

4. Select Lean Proteins: Acid reflux may be brought on by high-fat meats and dairy foods. Lean proteins, on the other hand, are easy on the stomach and less prone to create reflux symptoms. Examples of these include chicken, turkey, salmon, and tofu.

5. Select Whole Grains: Aiding in the alleviation of acid reflux symptoms, whole grains are an essential component of a balanced diet. Increase whole grains in your meals to help digestion and increase fiber, such as brown rice, quinoa, oats, and whole wheat bread.

6. Remain Hydrated with Water: Since water helps in digestion and lowers stomach acid, it is the optimal beverage option for you. You may minimize esophageal pain by avoiding acidic and carbonated liquids such as fizzy sodas and citrus juices.

7. Eat with Mindfulness: Slow, deliberate eating could minimize your probability of suffering symptoms of acid reflux. To improve good digestion and decrease reflux episodes, chew food fully, avoid eating while engaged or on the move, and sit upright when eating.

You may effectively comprehend the acid reflux diet and regulate the symptoms for improved digestive health by sticking to this advice and making intelligent food selections.

CUSTOMIZED MEAL PLANS

Personalized considerations must be addressed when establishing meal plans for persons with acid reflux. First, find out which foods are triggers and eliminate them. Lean meats, fruits, and vegetables should be your major sources of complete, low-acid diets. Reduce stomach discomfort and reduce overeating by combining smaller, more frequent meals.

To decide what is most comfortable for you, try alternative meal timings and amount levels. Stick to water and avoid away of carbonated or acidic beverages. Adopt mindful eating habits and nutritious grains to assist with digestion.

Tailored meal plans, with careful preparation and adjusting, may lessen symptoms of acid reflux and enhance your digestive health and overall well-being.

SECTION II: FUELING YOUR PATH TO WELL-BEING

BREAKFAST RECIPES

Sesame Pudding

Ingredients:

- 2 tsp. chia seeds

- 1/2 cup of unsweetened almond milk (or any other kind of milk)

- 1/4 teaspoon vanilla extract

- 1 teaspoon (optional) maple syrup or honey

- Fresh fruit (such as diced mango, berries, or sliced bananas) to serve as a topping

Instructions:

1. Place the chia seeds, almond milk, vanilla essence, and honey or maple syrup (if preferred) into a mixing bowl.

2. Give the mixture a vigorous swirl to make sure all of the chia seeds are incorporated.

3. To allow the chia seeds to absorb the liquid and thicken into a pudding-like consistency, cover the bowl and refrigerate for at least two hours, or better yet, overnight.

4. After the chia seed pudding has firmed, take it out of the fridge and properly combine it.

5. Distribute the pudding among serving jars or bowls.

6. Place your choice of fresh fruit on top of each plate.

7. Present cold and relish!

Prep Time: 5 minutes (plus chilling time)

Cooking Time: 0 minutes

Portion Size: 1 serving

Nutritional Information (per serving, excluding additional toppings):

- **Calories:** Approximately 120

- **Protein:** 4g

- **Fat:** 7g

- **Carbs:** 10g

- **Fiber:** 6g

- **Sugar:** 1g

- **Sodium:** Varies depending on ingredients

Allergy Information: If you pick a milk alternative other than almond milk, this recipe is free of nuts, dairy, and gluten. Those who are allergic to seeds, however, ought to keep away from chia seeds.

Tips for Acid Reflux Diet Plan:

- To decrease acidity and probable reflux triggers, use unsweetened almond milk or any other milk alternative without extra sugars.

If you would prefer not to have any added sugar or if you find that additional sweeteners make your reflux symptoms worse, then remove sweeteners like honey or maple syrup.

- To create diversity without boosting acidity, consider adding flavorings like cocoa powder or cinnamon.

- To further minimize acidity and probable reflux triggers, top the chia seed pudding with alkaline fruits like bananas, melons, or mangoes.

- To assess your tolerance, start with a tiny serving size. Chia seeds are heavy in fiber, therefore taking too much of them could induce discomfort in the digestive tract.

Veggie and Tomato Egg White Scramble

Ingredients:

- 4 beaten egg whites

- 1/2 cup chopped cherry tomatoes

- 1 teaspoon olive oil

- 1 cup fresh spinach leaves

- Season with salt and pepper.

Instructions:

1. In a nonstick skillet over medium heat, preheat the olive oil.

2. Include the chopped spinach in the pan and heat it for one to two minutes, or until it wilts.

3. Include the cherry tomatoes in the pan and cook until they start to soften, roughly one to two more minutes.

4. Cover the spinach and tomatoes in the pan with the egg whites.

5. Add salt and pepper to taste.

6. Gently scramble the egg whites with the vegetables using a spatula until they are well cooked, which should take 3–4 minutes.

7. Take the pan off of the burner after the egg whites are properly cooked.

8. Spoon the egg white scramble onto a dish and start serving straight immediately.

Prep Time: 5 minutes

Cooking Time: 5-7 minutes

Portion Size: 1 serving

Nutritional Information (per portion):

- **Calories:** Approximately 100

- **Protein:** 18g

- **Fat:** 2g

- **Carbohydrate:** 5g

- **Fiber:** 2g

- **Sugar:** 2g

- **Sodium:** Changes with the quantity of salt used

Allergy Information: This meal asks for eggs. This dinner should be avoided by anybody who is allergic to eggs. Those who are allergic to spinach or tomatoes should likewise avoid or use other acceptable substitutes for those components.

Tips for Acid Reflux Diet Plan:

- Since high-fat meals might worsen acid reflux symptoms, use egg whites instead of whole eggs to minimize the fat level.

- To lessen the likelihood of exacerbating acid reflux, cook using olive oil or other healthy fats rather than butter or heavy oils.

- Include foods that aren't acidic, such as tomatoes and spinach, since they are less prone to trigger reflux symptoms.

- Steer away from adding heavier or hotter toppings, such as cheese or spicy sauce, since these may worsen bouts of acid reflux.

- Present the egg white scramble over whole grain bread or a fruit side dish for a well-balanced meal that improves digestive well-being.

Oliver Quinoa Parfait

Ingredients:

- 1/2 cup of Greek yogurt

- 1/4 cup of granola (select low-fat, low-sugar variations)

- 1/4 cup of raw berries, such as raspberries, blueberries, or strawberries

- 1 tablespoon of optional honey for sweetness

Instructions:

1. Place half of the Greek yogurt in a serving glass or platter.

2. Sprinkle the yogurt layer with half of the granola.

3. Sprinkle the granola layer with half of the fresh berries.

4. Use the leftover Greek yogurt, granola, and berries to repeat the layers.

5. If you would like extra sweetness, sprinkle with honey.

6. Present right away and relish!

Prep Time: 5 minutes

Cooking Time: 0 minutes

Portion Size: 1 serving

Nutritional Information (per portion):

- **Calories:** Approximately 250

- **Protein:** 18g

- **Fat:** 6 g

- **Carbs:** 35g

- **Fiber:** 4g

- **Sugar:** 16g

- **Sodium:** Varies depending on ingredients

Allergy Information: If the granola is not gluten-free by certification, this recipe may have gluten in addition to dairy from Greek yogurt. Those with gluten or dairy sensitivity should use suitable replacements.

Tips for Acid Reflux Diet Plan:

- To decrease the likelihood of triggering acid reflux, choose plain Greek yogurt without any extra sugars or flavors.

- To lower fat content, which could worsen acid reflux symptoms, choose low-fat or non-fat Greek yogurt.

- Choose granola that has less added fat and sugar. Seek options that contain nuts, seeds, and whole grains for added minerals and fiber.

- To minimize added sugars and artificial additives, use fresh berries instead of canned or preserved fruits.

- Sliced bananas or peaches might be a nice substitute if berries are too acidic for your reflux.

Sweetheart Bowl

Ingredients:

- 1 frozen banana, chopped

- 1/2 cup of mixed frozen berries, including raspberries, blueberries, and strawberries

- 1/2 cup of Greek yogurt

- 1/4 cup almond milk, or any other kind of milk you want

- 1/3 cup of ground flaxseeds or chia seeds

- Optional toppings include granola, shredded coconut, nuts or seeds, honey, maple syrup, or sliced fresh fruit

Instructions:

1. Place frozen bananas, frozen mixed berries, Greek yogurt, almond milk, ground flaxseeds, or chia seeds in a blender.

2. Blend until smooth and creamy, adding extra almond milk as required to reach the consistency you desire.

3. Transfer the smoothie mix into a bowl.

4. Place your chosen fresh fruit slices, granola, shredded coconut, nuts, or seeds on top of the smoothie bowl. If you'd like, you may sprinkle some honey or maple syrup on top.

5. Present right away and relish!

Prep Time: 5 minutes

Cooking Time: 0 minutes

Portion Size: 1 serving

Nutritional Information (per dish, without toppings):

- **Calories:** 250

- **Protein:** 15g

- **Fat:** 5g

- **Carbs:** 40g

- **Fiber:** 8g

- **Sugar:** 20g

- **Sodium:** Varies depending on the ingredients

Allergy Information: Greek yogurt and almonds or seeds contain dairy in this meal. For people who are allergic to nuts or dairy, suitable replacements should be utilized.

Tips for Acid Reflux Diet Plan:

- To decrease the chance of triggering acid reflux, pick plain Greek yogurt without any extra sweeteners or flavors. If you would prefer not to have any added sugar or if you find that additional sweeteners make your reflux symptoms worse, then remove sweeteners like honey or maple syrup.

- Use alkaline fruits as a garnish, such as mangoes, bananas, or melons, to further minimize acidity and probable acid reflux reasons.

- When picking toppings, use low-acid choices such as unsweetened shredded coconut, pumpkin seeds, or sliced almonds.

- Try adding items like avocado or spinach to see if you can improve the nutrition and fiber content without increasing the acidity.

Cheese Pancakes

Ingredients:

- 1 cup of buckwheat flour

- 1 tablespoon of optional sugar or sweetness

- 1 tsp. baking powder

- 1/2 teaspoon of baking soda

- 1 cup milk (almond or oat milk works great)

- 1/4 teaspoon salt

- 1 large egg

- 2 tablespoons of melted oil (olive or coconut oil, for example) or butter

- More butter or oil to cook with

Instructions:

1. Combine the buckwheat flour, sugar (if using), baking soda, baking powder, and salt in a mixing bowl.

2. Beat the egg in another bowl, then add the milk and the melted oil or butter and stir.

3. Add the liquid components to the dry ingredients and stir just until mixed. The batter may be a bit lumpy; do not over-mix.

4. Give the mixture a 5- to 10-minute rest so that the baking soda and powder may become active.

5. Apply a small coating of oil or butter to a nonstick pan or griddle before heating it to medium heat.

6. Spoon each pancake's 1/4 cup of batter onto the pan.

7. After the pancake begins to bubble and its edges start to firm, flip it over and continue cooking it for a further one to two minutes, or until it becomes golden brown on both sides.

8. Repeat with the remaining batter, filling the pan with oil or butter as desired.

9. Top the pancakes with your choice of toppings and serve warm.

Prep Time: 10 minutes

Cooking Time: 10 minutes

Portion Size: Yields around 8 pancakes

Nutritional Information (per pancake):

- **Calories:** 120

- **Protein:** 4g

- **Fat:** 5g

- **Carbs:** 15g

- **Fiber:** 2g

- **Sugar:** 1g

- Sodium: 200mg

Allergy Information: Though it is a gluten-free grain, persons who are sensitive to gluten should ensure sure the buckwheat flour they use is certified gluten-free. If you use milk and eggs in this recipe, dairy is also included. For people who are allergic to eggs or dairy, suitable replacements should be utilized.

Tips for Acid Reflux Diet Plan:

- Choose unsweetened milk replacements, such as oat or almond milk, to minimize acidity.

- Avoid adding too much sugar, or if you do, use a tiny quantity of sweetener, as too much sugar could make acid reflux symptoms worse.

- Use alkaline fruits, such as sliced bananas or berries, on the pancakes rather than acidic ones, like citrus.

- For added nutrition and richness, sprinkle some honey or maple syrup over top, but use a dollop of Greek yogurt sparingly.

- Consume the pancakes in moderation, and monitor how much you consume to avoid overindulging, which may cause acid reflux.

Bowl of Quinoa Breakfast

Ingredients:

- 1/2 cup of quinoa

- 1 cup of water or milk (almond or oat milk works nicely here)

- 1/2 teaspoon of ground cinnamon

- 1 teaspoon of optionally sweet maple syrup or honey

- Fresh fruit (diced apples, berries, or sliced bananas) to serve as a topping

- Nuts or seeds (such as pumpkin seeds, walnuts, or almonds) for garnish

- Greek or coconut yogurt (optional) as a garnish

Instructions:

1. Rinse the quinoa in a fine-mesh strainer with cold water.

2. Combine the ground cinnamon, water, or milk, and rinsed quinoa in a small saucepan.

3. Once the mixture reaches a boiling point, turn down the heat to low and put a cover on the pot.

4. Simmer the quinoa for 15 to 20 minutes, or until it's mushy and all of the liquid has been absorbed.

5. Take the saucepan off of the flame when the quinoa is done, then use a fork to fluff the quinoa.

6. If using, mix in the maple syrup or honey.

7. Spoon cooked quinoa into each of the serving bowls.

8. Garnish each dish with nuts, seeds, and fresh fruit, along with Greek or coconut yogurt, if desired.

9. Enjoy and serve warm!

Prep Time: 5 minutes

Cooking Time: 15-20 minutes

Portion Size: 1 serving

Nutritional Information (per piece, without toppings):

- **Calories:** 220

- **Protein:** 8g

- **Fat:** 3g

- **Carbs:** 40g

- **Fiber:** 4g

- **Sugar:** 6g

- **Sodium:** 10mg

Allergy Information: Most persons with gluten sensitivity may safely consume quinoa since it is gluten-free. However, this dish should not be cooked by anybody who is allergic to quinoa.

Moreover, usual allergies include dairy (if using Greek yogurt) and almonds or seeds. If required, utilize suitable replacements.

Tips for Acid Reflux Diet Plan:

- Reduce acidity by using unsweetened milk alternatives, such as oat or almond milk.

- If you prefer a sugar-free alternative or if you find that sweets worsen your reflux symptoms, then avoid sweeteners like honey or maple syrup.

- Instead of using acidic fruits like citrus, use alkaline fruits as toppings, such as bananas, berries, or apples.

- For an added burst of protein and beneficial fats, consider almonds, walnuts, or pumpkin seeds, among other nuts and seeds.

- To decrease the likelihood of exacerbating acid reflux, choose basic Greek yogurts without extra sweeteners or flavors.

Oatmeal with Almond Butter and Banana

Ingredients:

- 1/2 cup of rolled oats

- 1 cup of milk or water (almond milk, for example)

- 1 ripe banana, chopped

- 1 tablespoon of almond butter

- If required sweetness, add honey or maple syrup

Instructions:

1. Bring the milk or water to a boil in a small saucepan.

2. Lower the heat to medium-low and mix in the rolled oats.

3. Simmer the oats for 5 to 7 minutes, stirring now and then, or until the consistency you desire is obtained.

4. Turn off the heat source and remove the pot off of the oats.

5. Place the prepared oats in a serving dish.

6. Add banana slices and almond butter on top of the cereal.

7. If desired, add a drizzle of honey or maple syrup for added sweetness.

8. Plate hot and relish!

Prep Time: 2 minutes

Cooking Time: 5 to 7 minutes

Portion Size: 1 serving

Nutritional Information (per portion):

- **Calories:** Approximately 300

- **Protein:** 8g

- **Fat:** 10g

- **Carbs:** 45g

- **Fiber:** 7g

- **Sugar:** 10g

- **Sodium:** Changes with the quantity of salt used

Allergy Information: Almonds and almond butter are used in this meal. If the oats are not gluten-free by certification, they might also contain gluten. Those with gluten or nut sensitivity should stay away from these items or use suitable replacements.

Tips for Acid Reflux Diet Plan:

- Choose almond milk without additional sugars to avoid exacerbating symptoms of acid reflux.

- Select ripe bananas; they will break down more readily and create less acid reflux.

- Make use of real almond butter that hasn't had any sugar or oil added.

- Try adding ground chia seeds or flaxseeds to deliver additional omega-3 fatty acids and fiber.

- Before serving, stir in a tiny quantity of yogurt or almond milk if you'd like it creamier.

INSPIRING QUOTES TO GET YOU ALONG WITH THE DIET

- "Feed your body, recuperate your soul."

Risotto with Brown Rice

Ingredients:

- 2 cups cooked brown rice

- 4 nori sheets

- 1/2 of a cucumber, chopped

- Slicing 1/2 of an avocado

- 1/2 of a carrot, chopped

- 1/2 julienned red bell pepper

- Tamari or soy sauce (optional) for dipping

- Wasabi and ginger pickles for presentation (optional)

Instructions:

1. Spread a sheet of nori seaweed on a newly cleaned kitchen towel or a bamboo sushi mat.

2. Evenly cover the nori seaweed with a thin layer of cooked brown rice, leaving a 1-inch border around the top edge.

3. Lay out the strips of red bell pepper, avocado, cucumber, and carrot across the middle of the rice.

4. Roll the rice and nori seaweed tightly around the filling, beginning at the bottom edge. Use a sushi mat or towel to aid the roll.

5. To seal the roll, dab a little water on the nori seaweed's top edge.

6. With the remaining nori seaweed sheets and filling ingredients, repeat the procedure.

7. Cut each sushi roll into 6–8 pieces using a sharp knife.

8. Present the sushi rolls with pickled ginger and wasabi, if preferred, and with soy sauce or tamari for dipping.

Prep Time: 20 minutes

Cooking Time: 0 minutes

Portion Size: 1 serving

Nutritional Information (per serving, excluding dipping sauce):

- **Calories:** Approximately 200

- **Protein:** 5g

- **Fat:** 5g

- **Carbs:** 35g

- **Fiber:** 5g

- **Sugar:** 2g

- **Sodium:** 200mg

Allergy Information: This recipe may be made vegan or vegetarian. On the other hand, anybody who is allergic to any of the compounds should avoid or use an acceptable replacement.

Tips for Acid Reflux Diet Plan:

- For extra fiber that may help in better digestion and lower the probability of reflux symptoms, consider brown rice rather than white rice.

- To avoid exacerbating acid reflux, keep clear of adding spicy ingredients to the sushi rolls, such as wasabi or sriracha.

- Accompany the sushi rolls with pickled ginger to help alleviate reflux symptoms and soothe the digestive system.

- Eat the sushi rolls in moderation; excessive intake could cause reflux. Be aware of food quantities.

Asparagus with Quinoa Salad

Ingredients:

- 1 cup of quinoa

- 2 cups of broth prepared with veggies or water

- 1/2 cup of cherry tomatoes

- 1 chopped cucumber

- Finely sliced 1/2 red onion

- 1/2 cup of chopped and pitted Kalamata olives

- 1/4 cup chopped fresh parsley

- Chopped 1/4 cup of fresh mint leaves

- 1/4 cup of optionally crumbled feta cheese

- Extra virgin olive oil, 2 teaspoons

- 1 tablespoon of vinegar prepared from red wine

- 1 minced clove of garlic

- Season with salt and pepper

- Optional serving of lemon wedges

Instructions:

1. Use a fine-mesh strainer to rinse the quinoa with cold water.

2. Quinoa and water or vegetable broth should be mixed in a medium-sized saucepan. Once the quinoa is cooked and the liquid has been absorbed, drop the heat to low, cover, and simmer for 15 to 20 minutes.

3. After the quinoa is done, pull it from the heat and let it cool a bit.

4. Combine the cooked quinoa, cherry tomatoes, cucumber, red onion, parsley, mint, and Kalamata olives in a large mixing bowl.

5. To produce the dressing, mix the extra virgin olive oil, red wine vinegar, minced garlic, salt, and pepper in a small bowl.

6. Toss the quinoa salad to ensure it is equally covered after adding the dressing.

7. Gently toss the salad one more after adding crumbled feta cheese, if using.

8. If desired, serve the chilled or room temperature Mediterranean quinoa salad with lemon wedges on the side for squeezing over the meal.

Prep Time: 10 minutes

Cooking Time: 15 to 20 minutes

Portion Size: 1 serving

Nutritional Information (per serving, sans feta cheese):

- **Calories:** Approximately 250

- **Protein:** 6g

- **Fat:** 10g

- **Carbs:** 35g

- **Fiber:** 5g

- **Sugar:** 3g

- **Sodium:** 300mg

Allergy Information: This recipe is vegetarian and free of gluten. On the other hand, anybody who is allergic to any of the compounds should avoid or use an acceptable replacement.

Tips for Acid Reflux Diet Plan:

- Swap the higher-fat or acidic grains like bulgur or couscous with quinoa as the base.

- To decrease acidity and probable acid reflux triggers, utilize alkaline foods like cucumber, cherry tomatoes, and red onion.

- If dairy aggravates your reflux symptoms, eliminate the feta cheese and use a dairy-free replacement instead.

- Employ extra virgin olive oil for the dressing as, in contrast to other oils, it is less likely to produce reflux.

- Savor the Mediterranean quinoa salad as a healthy and light meal that promotes digestion and minimizes the possibility of reflux symptoms. It is also strong in fiber.

Grilled Chicken Salad

Ingredients:

- 4 cups of various salad greens, such as arugula, spinach, or lettuce

- 1 boneless, skinless chicken breast

- 1/2 sliced cucumber

- 1/2 sliced bell pepper

- 1/2 cup of chopped cherry tomatoes

- Slicing 1/4 cup of red onion

- 2 tablespoons olive oil

- 1 tablespoon balsamic vinegar

- To taste, salt and pepper

Instructions:

1. Set the heat on your grill to medium-high.

2. Sprinkle salt and pepper on the chicken breast.

3. Cook the chicken breast on the grill for 6 to 8 minutes on each side, or until it's cooked through and no longer has a pink center.

4. Take the chicken off the grill and leave it a few minutes to rest before slicing it into thin strips.

5. Combine the mixed salad greens, bell pepper, cherry tomatoes, cucumber slices, and red onion slices in a large mixing dish.

6. To produce the dressing, combine the balsamic vinegar and olive oil in a small bowl.

7. Drizzle the salad components with the dressing, stirring to coat completely.

8. Arrange the salad mixture onto plates, then arrange the cooked chicken pieces on top.

9. Present right away and relish!

Prep Time: 10 minutes

Cooking Time: 12 to 16 minutes

Portion Size: 1 serving

Nutritional Information (per serving, without dressing):

- **Calories:** Approximately 250

- **Protein:** 25g

- **Fat:** 10g

- **Carbs:** 15g

- **Fiber:** 5g

- **Sugar:** 6g

- **Sodium:** 100 mg

Allergy Information: This meal asks for chicken. This dinner should be avoided by persons who are allergic to chicken. Anybody who is allergic to any of the components in the salad should also delete or substitute those parts appropriately.

Tips for Acid Reflux Diet Plan:

- Opt for lean chicken breast pieces; marinating the chicken in spicy or acidic sauces could increase symptoms of acid reflux.

- For the salad base, pick non-acidic vegetables like lettuce, bell pepper, and cucumber.

- Instead of creamy or acidic sauces, consider a simple dressing made with olive oil and balsamic vinegar. This may help avoid acid reflux.

- Use mild quantities of salt and pepper to season the salad instead of high-sodium spices, as this could aggravate acid reflux.

- Savor the salad as a well-balanced meal, with fiber from the vegetables and protein from the grilled chicken, which will aid with digestion and minimize the probability of acid symptoms.

Avocado with Salmon

Ingredients:

- 2 pieces of salmon and one bunch of trimmed asparagus

- 2 tablespoons of olive oil

- 1 sliced lemon

- Salt and pepper to taste

Instructions:

1. Turn the oven on to 400°F, or 200°C.

2. Transfer the asparagus trimmed to a baking sheet along with the salmon fillets.

3. Add salt and pepper for flavor, then pour over some olive oil. 4. Top the salmon with a layer of lemon slices.

5. Bake for 12 to 15 minutes in a preheated oven, or until the asparagus is tender and the salmon is cooked through.

6. Present right away and relish!

Prep Time: 5 minutes

Cooking Time: 12-15 minutes

Portion Size: 1 serving

Nutritional Information (per portion):

- **Calories:** Approximately 300

- **Protein:** 25g

- **Fat:** 18g

- **Carbohydrates:** 8g

- **Fiber:** 4g

- **Sugar:** 2g

- **Sodium:** 80mg

Allergy Information: There is seafood in this recipe—salmon. Those who are allergic to fish should not consume this dish. Additionally, persons who are allergic to any of the ingredients should avoid or use a suitable replacement for those goods.

Tips for Acid Reflux Diet Plan:

- For a lower-fat alternative that is healthier, go for fresh, wild-caught salmon instead of farmed salmon.

- Refrain from over-spicing or oil-consuming meals, as they may worsen the symptoms of acid reflux.

- To enhance digestion and add fiber, serve the salmon and asparagus with a side of quinoa or whole grain rice.

- Try adding herbs such as parsley or dill to enhance flavor without boosting the acidity.

Legumes with Turkey

Ingredients:

- Ground turkey: 1 pound

- Olive oil: 1 tablespoon

- Chopped garlic: 2 cloves

- 1 teaspoon of ground ginger

- 1/4 cup of soy sauce (gluten-free option: tamari)

- 1 tablespoon of vinegar prepared from rice

- 1 tsp. of maple syrup or honey

- 1 lettuce head with its leaves separated

- Topping possibilities include sliced bell peppers, sliced cucumbers, chopped green onions, and shredded carrots

Instructions:

1. Place olive oil in a pan and heat it to medium.

2. When the pan is fragrant, add the minced garlic and ground ginger and simmer for one to two minutes.

3. Add the ground turkey to the pan and heat, breaking it up with a spoon, until it is browned and cooked through.

4. Combine the rice vinegar, honey, maple syrup, and soy sauce in a small bowl.

5. Transfer the sauce to the pan with the cooked turkey and combine everything.

6. Simmer until the sauce gradually thickens, two to three minutes.

7. Spoon the mixture of turkey over the leaves of lettuce.

8. Add optional garnishes such as green onions, sliced bell peppers, cucumbers, and shredded carrots.

9. Immediately serve the lettuce wraps by wrapping up the leaves.

Prep Time: 10 minutes

Cooking Time: 15 minutes

Portion Size: 1 serving

Nutritional Information (per piece, eliminating optional toppings):

- **Calories:** Approximately 250

- **Protein:** 25g

- **Fat:** 15g

- **Carbohydrates:** 5g

- **Fiber:** 1g

- **Sugar:** 3g

- **Sodium:** 500mg

Allergy Information: Soy (found in soy sauce) is used in this meal. Those who are allergic to soy should use a soy-free replacement or avoid soy sauce completely. Additionally, persons who are allergic to any of the ingredients should avoid or use a suitable replacement for those goods.

Tips for Acid Reflux Diet Plan:

- Because high-fat meats may increase symptoms of acid reflux, use lean ground turkey to minimize the fat level.

- To limit your intake of salt, try tamari or low-sodium soy sauce. Using too much salt could increase reflux problems.

- To enhance digestion and add fiber, serve the turkey lettuce wraps with a side of steamed vegetables or a simple salad.

- If you're experiencing reflux troubles, consider preparing the wraps with iceberg or romaine lettuce leaves instead of more spicy greens like arugula or kale.

Cheese and Sweet Potato Stew

Ingredients:

- 2 medium sweet potatoes, chopped and peeling

- 1 canned (15 ounce) chickpeas, cleaned and drained

- 1 chopped onion

- 2 minced garlic cloves

- Diced tomatoes from 1 can (14.5 oz.)

- 2 cups vegetable broth

- 1 tsp. each of the ground cumin and coriander

- 1/2 tsp. paprika, smoked

- Salt and pepper to taste

- For garnish, add fresh parsley or cilantro (optional)

Instructions:

1. Drizzle some olive oil into a large skillet or Dutch oven and cook it over medium heat.

2. Cook the chopped onion for roughly five minutes, or until it turns soft.

3. Incorporate the finely chopped garlic, smoked paprika, ground coriander, and cumin. Sauté for one more minute, or until fragrant.

4. Pour the vegetable broth, diced tomatoes, chickpeas, and sweet potatoes into the saucepan. Mix thoroughly to combine.

5. Once the stew reaches a simmer, turn down the heat to low and cover it.

6. Until the sweet potatoes are tender, simmer the stew for 20 to 25 minutes.

7. Add pepper and salt according to taste.

8. Serve the stew hot, garnished with parsley or fresh cilantro, if desired.

Prep Time: 10 minutes

Cooking Time: 25 minutes

Portion Size: 1 serving

Nutritional Information (per portion):

- **Calories:** Approximately 300

- **Protein:** 10g

- **Fat:** 1g

- **Carbs:** 65g

- **Fiber:** 15g

- **Sugar:** 15g

- **Sodium:** 600mg

Allergy Information: This recipe may be made vegan or vegetarian. On the other hand, anybody who is allergic to any of the compounds should avoid or use an acceptable replacement.

Tips for Acid Reflux Diet Plan:

- To decrease the likelihood of producing reflux symptoms, consider low-acid products such as sweet potatoes and chickpeas.

- Steer away from adding acidic components to the stew, such as vinegar or citrus juice, since these could make acid reflux worse.

- To add fiber and assist in better digestion, serve the stew with whole grain bread or crackers.

- To boost the nutritional content of the stew, consider adding non-acidic greens like kale or spinach.

Vegetable Bowl with Quinoa

Ingredients:

- 1 cup quinoa

- 2 cups water or veggie broth

- 2 cups mixed vegetables, including broccoli, carrots, bell peppers, and zucchini

- 2 teaspoons of olive oil

- 1 teaspoon of dry herbs (oregano, rosemary, or thyme)

- Add salt and pepper to taste

- Add avocado slices, feta cheese (if vegan), and chopped fresh herbs as optional garnishes

Instructions:

1. Turn the oven on to 400°F, or 200°C.

2. Rinse the quinoa in a fine-mesh strainer with cold water.

3. Put the quinoa and water or vegetable broth in a medium-sized saucepan. Once the quinoa is cooked and the liquid has been absorbed, drop the heat to low, cover, and simmer for 15 to 20 minutes.

4. As the quinoa cooks, get the vegetables ready. Slicing them into tiny pieces, place them on a baking tray.

5. Add salt, pepper, and dried herbs to the vegetables after drizzling them with olive oil. Coat evenly by tossing.

6. Roast the vegetables for 20 to 25 minutes in a preheated oven, stirring them halfway through, or until they are tender and softly browned.

7. After the quinoa and vegetables have been cooked, spread them out among serving plates to create the bowls.

8. Add optional decorations, such as sliced avocado, freshly chopped fresh herbs, or crumbled feta cheese (if preferred).

9. Enjoy and serve warm!

Prep Time: 10 minutes

Cooking Time: 35-45 minutes

Portion Size: 1 serving

Nutritional Information (per piece, eliminating optional toppings):

- **Calories:** Approximately 300

- **Protein:** 8g

- **Fat:** 10g

- **Carbs:** 45g

- **Fiber:** 6g

- **Sugar:** 3g

- **Sodium:** 20mg

Allergy Information: This is a vegan and gluten-free dinner. Nevertheless, persons who are allergic to any of the vegetables should omit or use an adequate replacement.

Tips for Acid Reflux Diet Plan:

- For the roasted vegetable component, choose low-acid vegetables such as bell peppers, zucchini, carrots, and broccoli.

Refrain from putting acidic components in the cuisine, such as citrus or tomatoes, since these could increase symptoms of acid reflux.

- Avoid using spicy spices or sauces and stick to simple components like salt, pepper, and dry herbs.

- Add some avocado slices for healthy fats that might reduce stomach pain and minimize the possibility of reflux symptoms.

- Savor this healthy and well-balanced bowl of quinoa and roasted veggies as a meal that will help you digest food more efficiently and minimize the possibility of acid reflux attacks.

INSPIRING QUOTES TO GET YOU ALONG WITH THE DIET

- "Each bite could be a way towards wellness."

- "Let nourishment be thy medication and pharmaceutical be thy food."

- "Eat well, live well, and feel well."

- "Wellbeing isn't a goal, it's a journey."

- "You're what you eat, so eat well."

- "Awesome food is the establishment of veritable happiness."

- "Cooking is adore made self-evident."

- "Each recipe is a step towards a healthier you, a journey worth savoring."

- "In the kitchen, you're not just creating a meal, you're crafting a masterpiece of health and flavor."

- "Fuel your body with wholesome goodness, and watch it reciprocate with vitality."

DINNER RECIPES

Grilled Lemon and Dill Salmon

Ingredients:

- 2 fillets of salmon

- 1 slice of lemon

- 2 teaspoons finely chopped fresh dill

- Season with salt and pepper

Instructions:

1. Set the heat on your grill to medium-high.

2. On both sides, sprinkle salt and pepper onto the salmon fillets.

3. The salmon fillets should be cooked through and flaked easily with a fork after grilling for 4–5 minutes on each side.

4. Top each salmon fillet with a slice of lemon and some fresh dill during the last few minutes of cooking.

5. Take the salmon from the grill and serve right away.

Prep Time: 5 minutes

Cooking Time: 8-10 minutes

Portion Size: 1 serving

Nutritional Information (per portion):

- **Calories:** Approximately 250

- **Protein:** 25g

- **Fat:** 15g

- **Carbohydrates:** 1g

- **Fiber:** 0g

- **Sugar:** 0g

- **Sodium:** Changes according to the spice

Allergy Information: Salmon, a kind of fish, is used in this dish. Those who are allergic to fish should not eat this meal. Additionally, people who are allergic to any of the substances should avoid or use an appropriate alternative for those products.

Tips for Acid Reflux Diet Plan:

- For a healthier alternative with less fat, go for fresh salmon instead of farmed salmon.

- Steer clear of too much seasoning or marinades; substances that are heavy in fat or acid might aggravate symptoms of acid reflux.

To aid in improved digestion and lessen the chance of reflux symptoms, serve the grilled salmon with non-acidic side dishes like quinoa or steamed vegetables.

- Eat the grilled salmon in moderation; watch portion sizes to prevent overindulging, which can aggravate reflux.

Baked Herb-Crusted Chicken Breast

Ingredients:

- 2 skinless, boneless chicken breasts

- 2 teaspoons of olive oil

- Minced 2 cloves of garlic

- 1 tsp. of dried thyme

- 1 teaspoon of rosemary, dried

- 1 teaspoon of dehydrated oregano

- Season with salt and pepper

- Optional serving of lemon wedges

Instructions:

1. Start the oven at 400°F or 200°C.

2. Olive oil, minced garlic, dried thyme, dried rosemary, and dried oregano should all be combined in a small bowl.

3. Season the chicken breasts on both sides with salt and pepper and transfer them to a baking dish.

4. Evenly coat the chicken breasts by brushing them with the herb and olive oil mixture.

5. Bake the chicken for 20 to 25 minutes, or until it is cooked through and reaches an internal temperature of 165°F (75°C), in a preheated oven.

6. Before serving, take the chicken out of the oven and allow it to rest for a few minutes.

7. If desired, serve the baked chicken breast with lemon wedges on the side for you to squeeze over the chicken.

Prep Time: 10 minutes

Cooking Time: 20 to 25 minutes

Portion Size: 1 serving

Nutritional Information (per portion):

- **Calories:** Approximately 250

- **Protein:** 25g

- **Fat:** 15g

- **Carbohydrates:** 0g

- **Fiber:** 0g

- **Sugar:** 0g

- **Sodium:** Changes according to the spice

Allergy Information: This recipe does not contain dairy or gluten. On the other hand, anyone who is allergic to any of the substances should avoid or use an appropriate alternative.

Tips for Acid Reflux Diet Plan:

- Usc skinless, lean chicken breasts to cut down on fat content, as high-fat meats can aggravate symptoms of acid reflux.

- Add flavor with herbs such as thyme, rosemary, and oregano; avoid adding acidity, as acidic ingredients can aggravate reflux.

- To improve digestion and lessen the chance of reflux symptoms, serve the baked chicken breast with non-acidic side dishes like brown rice or roasted vegetables.

- Take care of portion sizes and enjoy the baked chicken breast in moderation to prevent overindulging, which can aggravate reflux.

Pesto-Crusted Zucchini Noodles

Ingredients:

- 2 medium zucchini

- 1/4 cup basil pesto

- 1/2 cherry tomatoes, if desired, for garnish

- Grated Parmesan cheese, if desired, as a garnish

- Pine nuts, if desired, as a garnish

Instructions:

1. Remove the ends from the zucchinis and wash them.

2. Slice the zucchini into thin strips and use a spiralizer or vegetable peeler to make zucchini noodles.

3. After heating a sizable skillet to medium heat, add the zucchini noodles.

4. Cook, stirring occasionally, until the zucchini noodles are heated through but still crisp-tender, 2 to 3 minutes.

5. After turning off the stove, remove the skillet from the heat and toss the zucchini noodles in the pesto until well-coated.

6. Optional garnishes for the zucchini noodles include pine nuts, grated Parmesan cheese, and cherry tomatoes.

Prep Time: 10 minutes

Cooking Time: 30 minutes

Portion Size: 1 serving

Nutritional Informational (per serving, without optional garnishes):

- **Calories:** Approximately 150

- **Protein:** 4g

- **Fat:** 12g

- **Carbohydrates:** 8g

- **Fiber:** 2g

- **Sugar:** 4g

- **Sodium:** 200mg

Allergy Information: This is a vegetarian recipe. But those who are allergic to nuts should substitute another type of nut in place of the pine nuts. Additionally, people who are allergic to any of the substances should avoid or use an appropriate alternative for those products.

Tips for Acid Reflux Diet Plan:

- To lessen the possibility of aggravating reflux symptoms, use store-bought or homemade low-acid pesto.

- To preserve the crisp-tender texture of the zucchini noodles, avoid overcooking them. Overcooked vegetables can worsen acid reflux.

- Serve the zucchini noodles with lean protein sources, such as shrimp or grilled chicken, to create a well-balanced meal that lessens the chance of reflux symptoms and improves digestion.

- Eat the zucchini noodles in moderation; if you overeat, it can aggravate reflux. Be mindful of portion sizes.

Veggie Stir-Fry with Turkey

Ingredients:

- 1 tablespoon of olive oil

- 1 pound of turkey meat

- 2 cups of mixed veggies, including snap peas, carrots, bell peppers, and broccoli

- Minced 2 cloves of garlic

- 2 teaspoons of soy sauce or low-sodium tamari

- 1 tablespoon of vinegar made from rice

- 1 tsp. Honey, also known as maple syrup

- 1 tsp. of finely grated ginger

- Ready to serve cooked quinoa or brown rice

Instructions:

1. In a big wok or skillet, warm up the olive oil over medium-high heat.

2. Using a spoon, break up the cooked ground turkey as it browns in the skillet.

3. Add the minced garlic and mixed vegetables to the skillet. The vegetables should be crisp-tender after 5 to 6 minutes of stir-frying.

4. Mix the rice vinegar, soy sauce, grated ginger, honey, or maple syrup in a small bowl.

5. Cover the veggies and turkey in the skillet with the sauce. Coat evenly by stirring to combine.

6. After two to three more minutes of cooking, the sauce should have somewhat thickened.

7. Overcooked brown rice or quinoa, serve the turkey and vegetable stir-fry hot.

Prep Time: 10 minutes

Cooking Time: 15 minutes

Portion Size: 1 serving

Nutritional Information (per serving, omitting quinoa and rice):

- **Calories:** Approximately 250

- **Protein:** 25g

- **Fat:** 10g

- **Carbs:** 15g

- **Fiber:** 5g

- **Sugar:** 8g

- **Sodium:** 400mg

Allergy Information: This recipe contains no dairy or gluten. For those who are allergic to soy, a soy-free substitute for tamari or soy sauce should be used. Additionally, people who are allergic to any of the substances should avoid or use an appropriate alternative for those products.

Tips for Acid Reflux Diet Plan:

- To lower the fat content, use lean ground turkey rather than higher-fat meats, as high-fat foods can aggravate the symptoms of acid reflux.

- Select non-acidic veggies for the stir-fry, such as carrots, broccoli, and bell peppers, to lessen the possibility of bringing on reflux symptoms.

- Choose tamari or low-sodium soy sauce to reduce your intake of sodium because too much salt can aggravate reflux.

- Serve the cooked brown rice or quinoa alongside the turkey and vegetable stir-fry to improve digestion and add extra fiber, which will lessen the chance of reflux symptoms.

Puffed Bell Peppers with Quinoa

Ingredients:

- 4 bell peppers (of any hue), with the seeds and tops removed

- 1 cup rinsed quinoa

- 2 cups of broth made of vegetables

- 1 (15-oz) can of black beans, washed and drained

- 1 cup of corn kernels, either canned, frozen, or fresh

- Diced tomatoes (either fresh or canned), 1 cup

- Diced onion, 1/2 cup

- Minced 2 cloves of garlic

- 1 tsp. of ground cumin

- 1 teaspoon of chili powder

- Season with salt and pepper

- Adding shredded cheese, avocado slices, or chopped cilantro as garnish is optional.

Instructions:

1. Set oven temperature to 375°F or 190°C.

2. Combine the vegetable broth and quinoa in a medium-sized saucepan. Once the quinoa is cooked and the liquid has been absorbed, decrease the heat to low, cover, and simmer for 15 to 20 minutes.

3. Add the cooked quinoa, black beans, corn kernels, diced tomatoes, diced onion, minced garlic, ground cumin, chili powder, salt, and pepper to a large mixing bowl.

4. Mix the quinoa mixture thoroughly with a fork.

5. Gently press down to fill each bell pepper to the brim with the quinoa mixture.

6. The filled bell peppers should be put in a baking dish and covered with aluminum foil.

7. Bake for 25 to 30 minutes, or until the bell peppers are soft, in an oven that has been preheated.

8. To allow the tops to brown slightly, remove the foil during the final five minutes of baking.

9. Serve the bell peppers with quinoa stuffing hot, garnished with extras if preferred.

Prep Time: 15 minutes

Cooking Time: 45 to 60 minutes

Portion Size: 1 filled bell pepper

Nutritional Information (per stuffed bell pepper, no toppings):

- **Calories:** Approximately 300

- **Protein:** 12g

- **Fat:** 2g

- **Carbs:** 60g

- **Fiber:** 12g
- **Sugar:** 8g
- **Sodium:** 600mg

Allergy Information: This dish may be made vegan or vegetarian. On the other hand, anyone who is allergic to any of the substances should avoid or use an appropriate alternative.

Tips for Acid Reflux Diet Plan:
- To lessen the chance of inducing reflux symptoms, opt for low-acid ingredients like bell peppers, quinoa, and black beans.
Steer clear of adding hot seasonings or toppings as they may worsen acid reflux.
- To improve digestion and add fiber, serve the quinoa-stuffed bell peppers with a side of steamed vegetables or a straightforward salad.
- Eat the stuffed bell peppers as a nutritious, well-balanced meal to improve digestion and lessen the chance of reflux symptoms. They are also high in fiber.

Sweethearts Baked with Greek Yogurt

Ingredients:

- 2 medium sweet potatoes

- 1/2 cup Greek yogurt

- 1 tsp. of maple syrup or honey

- Optional cinnamon garnish

Instructions:

1. Start the oven at 400°F or 200°C.

2. After washing, make several fork piercings in the sweet potatoes.

3. After placing the sweet potatoes on a baking sheet, bake them in the preheated oven for 45 to 60 minutes, or until a fork inserted into them comes out tender.

4. After taking them out of the oven, allow the sweet potatoes to cool slightly.

5. Use a fork to fluff the insides of each sweet potato after cutting it in half lengthwise.

6. Combine the Greek yogurt and maple syrup or honey in a small bowl.

7. Onto each half of a sweet potato, spoon some Greek yogurt that has been sweetened.

8. If desired, garnish with a sprinkle of cinnamon.

9. Serve the sweet potatoes hot from the oven.

Prep Time: 5 minutes

Cooking Time: 45-60 minutes

Portion Size: 1/2 sweet potato

Nutritional Information (per serving):
- **Calories:** Approximately 200
- **Protein:** 8g
- **Fat:** 0g
- **Carbohydrates:** 40g
- **Fiber:** 6g
- **Sugar:** 12g
- **Sodium:** 50mg

Allergy Information: This recipe is gluten-free. However, individuals with dairy allergies should omit Greek yogurt or use a dairy-free alternative. Additionally, individuals with allergies to any of the ingredients should omit or substitute those ingredients accordingly.

Tips for Acid Reflux Diet Plan:
- Opt for plain Greek yogurt instead of flavored ones for the topping as the latter may worsen acid reflux by including additional sugars or flavorings with strong acids.
- Steer clear of acidic toppings like tomatoes or citrus as they may exacerbate reflux problems.

- To balance the meal and aid in improved digestion, serve the baked sweet potatoes with a small quantity of lean protein or a side of non-acidic veggies.

- Savor the baked sweet potatoes as a filling and high-nutrient choice for those on an acid-reflux diet.

Spinach Lentil Soup

Ingredients:

- 1 cup of washed dry lentils

- 4 cups of broth made with vegetables

- 1 chopped onion

- 2 minced garlic cloves

- 2 diced carrots

- 2 chopped celery stalks

- 1 (14.5-oz) can of chopped tomatoes

- 2 cups of raw spinach

- 1 teaspoon of thyme, dried

- 1 teaspoon of oregano, dried

- To taste, add salt and pepper

Instructions:

1. The vegetable broth and dry lentils should be combined in a big saucepan.

2. After bringing to a boil, lower the heat to a simmer and cook for 20 to 25 minutes, or until the lentils are soft.

3. Heat a sprinkle of olive oil in a different skillet over medium heat.

4. To the pan, add the diced onion, diced carrots, diced celery, and minced garlic. Simmer the veggies for five to six minutes, or until they are tender.

5. Toss the cooked veggies into the lentil pot.

6. Add the dried oregano, dry thyme, and chopped tomatoes with their juices.

7. To let the flavors combine, simmer the soup for a further 10 to 15 minutes.

8. Once the spinach has wilted, simmer it for a further two to three minutes after stirring in the new leaves.

9. To taste, add more salt and pepper to the lentil soup.

10. Warm lentil soup should be served.

Prep Time: 10 minutes

Cooking Time: 35 to 40 minutes

Portion Size: 1 cup

Nutritional Information (per serving):

- **Calories:** Approximately 200

- **Protein:** 12g

- **Fat:** 1g

- **Carbohydrates:** 35g

- **Fiber:** 15g

- **Sugar:** 6g

- **Sodium:** 700mg

Allergy Information: This dish is vegan and vegetarian. Those who are allergic to any of the components, however, should omit or use an appropriate alternative.

Tips for Acid Reflux Diet Plan:

- Protein and fiber from lentils are excellent for digestion and can help lessen acid reflux symptoms. Including lentil soup in your diet may provide you with a filling, healthy meal that is easy on the stomach.

- Refrain from including acidic components in the lentil soup, such as vinegar or lemon juice, as they might aggravate symptoms of acid reflux. Rather, add herbs and spices like black pepper, oregano, and thyme to the soup.

- Rich in vitamins and minerals, spinach is a non-acidic leafy green. The lentil soup gains more minerals and fiber from the addition of spinach without becoming more acidic. To make the spinach simpler to digest, make sure it's cooked all the way through.

- To add texture and taste, serve the lentil soup as a stand-alone dish or with a side salad or a slice of whole grain bread. Pay attention to portion proportions to avoid overindulging, which can aggravate acid reflux.

- Savor the lentil soup as a filling and cozy meal that complements your acid reflux diet plan, offers vital nutrients, and helps maintain the health of your digestive system.

INSPIRING QUOTES TO GET YOU ALONG WITH THE DIET

- "Savor the flavors of healing."

- "Eating sound could be a self-respect."

- "The secret ingredient in every recipe is the commitment to your well-being."

- "In the kitchen, you hold the paintbrush to create your masterpiece on the canvas of health."

- "Cooking is a mindful act of self-love; each recipe is a chapter in your wellness story."

- "Flavorful meals are the roadmap to a healthier, happier you; let the journey begin in your kitchen."

- "In the kitchen, you have the power to transform ingredients into a symphony of health and joy."

- "Savor the taste of good health; it's the most delicious choice you'll ever make."

- "Cook with intention; each recipe is a step towards a healthier, more vibrant version of you."

- "Celebrate the joy of eating well; every bite is a dance of flavors on the palate of life."

Sweetheart Potato Fries Baked

Ingredients:

- 2 medium sweet potatoes, chopped into fries after peeling

- 1 tablespoon of olive oil

- To taste, add salt and pepper

Instructions:

1. Set the oven temperature to 425°F (220°C).

2. Toss the sweet potato fries with salt, pepper, and olive oil in a wide bowl until they are fully coated.

3. Place the fries on a parchment paper-lined baking sheet in a single layer.

4. Bake for 25 to 30 minutes in a preheated oven, flipping the fries halfway through, or until they are crispy and have a golden brown hue.

5. Take out of the oven and serve immediately away.

Prep Time: 10 minutes

Cooking Time: 25 to 30 minutes

Portion Size: 1 medium sweet potato

Nutritional Information (per medium plate of sweet potatoes):

- **Calories:** Approximately 150

- **Protein:** 2g

- **Fat:** 4g

- **Carbohydrates:** 27g

- **Fiber:** 4g

- **Sugar:** 6g

- **Sodium:** 200mg

Allergy Information: There is no dairy or gluten in this dish. Those who are sensitive to sweet potatoes or olive oil, however, should stay away from this meal. Those who are allergic to any of the compounds should also omit or use an acceptable replacement.

Tips for Acid Reflux Diet Plan:

- Sweet potatoes are a low-acid food that may help patients with GERD feel better. Baking them instead of frying them reduces unnecessary fat and probable allergies.

- Steer away from adding cayenne pepper chili powder or other acidic spices to the fries as they may make GERD symptoms worse.

- Eat the sweet potato fries in moderation and be aware of quantity sizes, as overindulging in them could worsen acid reflux patients' pain.

- To add flavor and nutrition, serve the fries with a side of hummus prepared with just two ingredients or a non-acidic dipping sauce.

Hydro-Trail Mix DIY

Ingredients:

- 1 cup of almonds, unsalted
- 1 cup of cashews, unsalted
- 1/2 cup of pumpkin seeds
- 1/2 cup of unsweetened dried cranberries
- 1/2 cup of dark chocolate chips, if desired

Instructions:

1. Almonds, cashews, pumpkin seeds, dried cranberries, and dark chocolate chips (if used) should all be mixed in a large mixing bowl.
2. Mix the ingredients until they are all distributed evenly.
3. For simple grab-and-go snacks, separate the trail mix into individual snack bags or keep it in an airtight container.

Prep Time: 5 minutes
Cooking Time: 30 seconds
Portion Size: 1/4 cup

Nutritional Information (per 1/4 cup portion):

- **Calories:** Approximately 200

- **Protein:** 6g

- **Fat:** 15g

- **Carbohydrates:** 15g

- **Fiber:** 3g

- **Sugar:** 8g

- **Sodium:** 0mg

Allergy Information: There are nuts in this recipe. Those who are allergic to nuts should replace alternative components or leave out the nuts. Those who are allergic to any of the compounds should also omit or use an acceptable replacement.

Tips for Acid Reflux Diet Plan:

- Select unsalted nuts and seeds to decrease your intake of sodium since too much salt could make your symptoms of acid reflux worse.

- Choose unsweetened dried cranberries to keep away from added sweets, since they could worsen reflux.

- You may substitute the dark chocolate chips with carob chips if you have GERD that is worsened by chocolate.

- Divide up the trail mix into tiny parts to prevent overindulging, which may worsen GERD symptoms.

- Savor the trail mix as a full and wholesome snack that offers you energy and important nutrients all day long.

Strawberry-Banana Drink

Ingredients:

- 1 mature banana

- 1/2 cup frozen or fresh blueberries

- 1/2 cup of Greek yogurt

- 1/2 cup non-dairy milk, such as almond milk.

- 1 tablespoon (optional) of maple syrup or honey

- Ice cubes, if desired

Instructions:

1. After peeling, place the banana in a blender.

2. To the blender, add the blueberries, Greek yogurt, almond milk, and, if preferred, honey or maple syrup.

3. To make the smoothie colder, feel free to add a few ice cubes to the blender.

4. Blend until creamy and smooth.

5. After pouring the smoothie into glasses, serve it immediately away.

Prep Time: 5 minutes

Cooking Time: 0 minutes

Portion Size: 1 portion

Nutritional Information (per serving):

- **Calories:** Approximately 200

- **Protein:** 8g

- **Fat:** 3g

- **Carbohydrates:** 40g

- **Fiber:** 5g

- **Sugar:** 25g

- **Sodium:** 100mg

Allergy Information: Greek yogurt, a dairy product, is used in this recipe. Those who are allergic to dairy products should replace a dairy-free alternative or omit Greek yogurt. Those who are allergic to any of the compounds should also omit or use an acceptable replacement.

Tips for Acid Reflux Diet Plan:

- To have a naturally sweet taste without added sweeteners that irritate acid reflux symptoms, pick ripe bananas and fresh blueberries.

- Choose plain Greek yogurt instead of flavors or added sugars that could irritate reflux. Additionally, Greek yogurt includes less lactose than typical yogurt, which helps some individuals digest it more readily.

- You may use almond milk or any other non-dairy milk alternative in the smoothie if dairy affects your reflux symptoms.

- Savor the blueberry banana smoothie as a light and healthy breakfast or snack that is easy on the stomach and could help lessen symptoms of acid reflux.

Rice Cake with Banana Slices and Almond Butter

Ingredients:

- 1 rice cake
- 1 tablespoon of almond butter
- 1/2 banana, sliced

Instructions:

1. Evenly apply almond butter over the rice cake.

2. Put the banana slices in an arrangement over the almond butter.

3. Serve straight away.

Prep Time: 2 minutes

Cooking Time: 0 minutes

Portion Size: 1 portion

Nutritional Information (per serving):

- **Calories:** Approximately 150

- **Protein:** 3g

- **Fat:** 7g

- **Carbohydrates:** 19g

- **Fiber:** 3g

- **Sugar:** 6g

- **Sodium:** 0mg

Allergy Information: Almonds are included in this dish. Those who are allergic to nuts should not cook this meal. Those who are allergic to any of the compounds should also omit or use an acceptable replacement.

Tips for Acid Reflux Diet Plan:

- For persons with acid reflux, rice cakes are a low-acid option for bread or crackers that may be gentler to their digestive systems.

- Almond butter is a fantastic source of protein and healthy fats, however, people who suffer acid reflux should stick to natural almond butter that doesn't contain any added salt or sugar.

- Because they contain less acid and may counteract stomach acid, bananas are a healthy fruit alternative for persons who suffer acid reflux.

- Savor the rice cake with sliced banana and nut butter for a simple, light lunch or snack that is easy on the stomach and could help lessen symptoms of acid reflux.

Ginger Turmeric Tea

Ingredients:

- 2 cups of water

- 1-inch piece of young ginger, daintily sliced

- 1 teaspoon of ground turmeric

- 1 tablespoon of honey (optional, for sweetness)

- Juice from 1/2 a lemon (optional, for extra taste)

Instructions:

1. In a small pan, heat the water to a bubble over medium temperature.

2. Add the sliced ginger and ground turmeric to the boiling water.

3. Diminish the warm to moo and allow the mix to stew for approximately 5 minutes.

4. Remove the pot from the heat and let the tea steep for a further 5 minutes.

5. Strain the tea into cups using a fine-mesh strainer or cheesecloth.

6. Stir in honey and lemon juice, if preferred, for sweetness and flavor.

7. Serve the tea hot and enjoy!

Prep Time: 5 minutes

Cooking Time: 10 minutes

Portion Size: Makes 2 servings

Nutritional Information (per serving):

- **Calories:** 15

- **Carbohydrates:** 4 g

- **Fat:** 0 g

- **Protein:** 0 g

- **Fiber:** 0 g

- **Sugars:** 3 g

- Sodium: 0 mg

Allergy Information: This dish is naturally gluten-free, dairy-free, and nut-free. However, anyone with sensitivities to ginger or turmeric should avoid this tea or contact with their healthcare professional before ingesting it.

Tips for Acid Reflux Diet Plan:

- Use fresh ginger and turmeric whenever feasible for optimal taste and health benefits.

- Adjust the quantity of honey and lemon juice according to your taste preferences and tolerance for acidity.

- Allow the tea to cool somewhat before consuming to minimize any discomfort to the throat and esophagus.

- Sip the tea slowly and deliberately, relishing each relaxing sip and letting the ingredients work their magic on your digestive system.

- Incorporate this tea into your daily routine as a peaceful and therapeutic beverage to help ease symptoms of acid reflux and support overall digestive health.

Enjoy this comfortable Ginger Turmeric Tea as a relaxing supplement to your Acid Reflux Diet Plan!

2-Ingredient Hummus

Ingredients:

- 1 (15-oz) can of rinsed and drained chickpeas

- 2 tablespoons of tahini

Instructions:

1. Place the rinsed and drained chickpeas and tahini in a food processor.

2. Blend until creamy and smooth, pausing periodically to scrape down the bowl's edges.

3. Add a tablespoon of water at a time to the hummus if it's too thick until you reach the correct consistency.

4. After transferring the hummus to a serving dish, you may optionally sprinkle it with olive oil.

5. Accompany with rice cakes, whole grain crackers, or vegetable sticks.

Prep Time: 5 minutes

Cooking Time: 30 seconds

Portion Size: 2 tablespoons

Nutritional Information (per serving of 2 tablespoons):

- **Calories:** Approximately 70

- **Protein:** 3g

- **Fat:** 4g

- **Carbohydrates:** 6g

- **Fiber:** 2g

- **Sugar:** 0g

- **Sodium:** 60mg

Allergy Information: Tahini contains sesame, which is used in this dish. This meal should not be cooked by anybody who is allergic to sesame. Those who are allergic to any of the compounds should also omit or use an acceptable replacement.

Tips for Acid Reflux Diet Plan:

- Tahini is a fantastic source of heart-healthy fats and may benefit those who experience acid reflux. However, because high-fat meals may increase symptoms, portion control is key.

- Savor the hummus as a dip for low-acid fresh vegetables like bell peppers, carrots, and cucumbers, which may help lessen reflux symptoms.

- Steer away from adding acidic components to the hummus, such as garlic or lemon juice, as they could worsen reflux.

- Include hummus in your diet cautiously since excessive consumption could cause discomfort for individuals who have acid reflux.

INSPIRING QUOTES TO GET YOU ALONG WITH THE DIET

- "Eat well, live fully."

- "Food is fuel for your body and soul."

- "Eating sound could be a self-respect."

- "Back your body what it merits."

- "Wellness begins on your plate."

- "The primary niche is health."

- "Mending starts with what you put on your plate."

- "Treat your body like a sanctuary, nourish it with love."

VEGETARIAN RECIPES

Rice with Baked Chicken Thighs

Ingredients:

- 4 skin-on, bone-in chicken thighs

- 1 cup of white long-grain rice

- 2 cups of chicken stock

- 1 tablespoon of olive oil

- To taste, add salt and pepper

- Optional: your preferred herbs and spices (garlic powder, paprika, thyme)

Instructions:

1. Turn the oven on to 375°F, or 190°C.

2. Salt, pepper, and any additional herbs or spices can be used to season the chicken thighs.

3. In an oven-safe pan, warm the olive oil over medium-high heat.

4. For five to six minutes, or until golden brown, sear the chicken thighs skin-side down.

5. After 3-4 minutes, turn the chicken thighs over and brown the other side.

6. After removing them from the pan, set the chicken thighs aside.

7. Stir together the rice and chicken broth after adding them to the pan.

8. Reintroduce the chicken thighs skin-side up over the rice in the skillet.

9. Place a lid or piece of aluminum foil over the skillet and place it in the oven that has been preheated.

10. Bake for 35 to 40 minutes, or until the rice is soft and the chicken is cooked through.

11. Take it out of the oven and give it a five-minute rest before serving.

12. Overheated rice, serve the roasted chicken thighs.

Prep Time: 10 minutes

Cooking Time: 45 to 50 minutes

Portion Size: 1 chicken thigh paired with rice

Nutritional Information (per serving):

- **Calories:** Approximately 400

- **Protein:** 25g

- **Fat:** 15g

- **Carbohydrates:** 35g

- **Fiber:** 1g

- **Sugar:** 0g

- **Sodium:** 500mg

Allergy Information: There is no gluten in this recipe. Those who are allergic to chicken or any other component, however, should delete or use an acceptable replacement.

Tips for Acid Reflux Diet Plan:

- To boost flavor and moisture, pick bone-in, skin-on chicken thighs; however, remove the skin before eating to minimize the fat content, since high-fat meals might worsen acid symptoms.

- Instead of brown rice, try long-grain white rice, which contains less fiber and might be easier for individuals with acid reflux to digest.

- Savor the roasted chicken thighs over rice as a well-balanced entrée that is easy on the stomach and abundant in protein, carbohydrates, and vital nutrients.

Bars of Bananas

Ingredients:

- 2 mashed, ripe bananas

- 1 cup of rolled oats

- 1/4 cup chopped nuts, such as almonds or walnuts

- 1/4 cup dried cranberries or raisins

- 1 tablespoon (optional) of maple syrup or honey

- 1 teaspoon of cinnamon

- 1 dash of salt

Instructions:

1. Preheat the oven to 350°F (175°C).

2. Mashed bananas, rolled oats, chopped nuts, raisins or dried cranberries, cinnamon, salt, and honey or maple syrup (if desired) should all be put in a mixing bowl. To make sure all the ingredients are evenly combined, give it a vigorous stir.

3. Spread the ingredients evenly in a baking dish that has been greased or lined with parchment paper.

4. Bake for 20 to 25 minutes in a preheated oven, or until the bars are firm to the touch and the edges are golden brown.

5. Take it out of the oven and allow it to cool entirely before slicing it into bars.

6. After chilling, cut into bars and refrigerate for up to a week in an airtight container.

Prep Time: 10 minutes

Cooking Time: 20 to 25 minutes

Portion Size: 1 bar

Nutritional Information (for Each Bar):

- **Calories:** Approximately 100

- **Protein:** 3g

- **Fat:** 3g

- **Carbohydrates:** 18g

- **Fiber:** 2g

- **Sugar:** 7g

- **Sodium:** 0mg

Allergy Information: There are nuts in this recipe. Those who are allergic to nuts should replace alternative components or leave out the nuts. Those who are allergic to any of the compounds should also omit or use an acceptable replacement.

Tips for Acid Reflux Diet Plan:

- Select ripe bananas to enjoy their intrinsic sweetness without the added sugars that increase acid reflux symptoms.

- Choose dried fruits without added sugars, such as cranberries or raisins, since they could irritate reflux.

- Savor the banana bars as a heart-healthy snack or breakfast option that may help lessen symptoms of acid reflux.

Verdant Smoothie

Ingredients:

- 1 cup of raw spinach

- 1/2 cup of thinly chopped cucumber

- 1/2 banana

- 1/2 cup of verdejos

- 1/2 cup of almond milk without sugar

- 1 tablespoon (optional) of maple syrup or honey

Instructions:

1. In a blender, add the chopped cucumber, banana, green grapes, fresh spinach leaves, and almond milk.

2. Add additional honey or maple syrup for sweetness, if you'd like.

3. Blend until creamy and smooth.

4. Serve the green smoothie straight soon after putting it into glasses.

Prep Time: 5 minutes

Cooking Time: 0 minutes

Portion Size: 1 portion

Nutritional Information (per serving):

- **Calories:** Approximately 120

- **Protein:** 2g

- **Fat:** 2g

- **Carbohydrates:** 25g

- **Fiber:** 4g

- **Sugar:** 17g

- **Sodium:** 100mg

Allergy Information: There is no dairy or gluten in this dish. Those who are allergic to any of the components, however, should omit or use an acceptable replacement.

Tips for Acid Reflux Diet Plan:

- People with acid reflux may gain relief from their symptoms by consuming green smoothies that include non-acidic fruits and vegetables such as spinach, cucumber, and green grapes.

- Citrus fruits, such as oranges or grapefruits, should not be added to the smoothie since they may make reflux symptoms worse.

- Choose unsweetened almond milk to prevent excessive sugar consumption, since it may irritate reflux.

- Savor the green smoothie as a hydrating and nutrient-dense breakfast or snack that offers you the vitamins and minerals you need to support your acid reflux diet plan.

Sandwich with Peanut Butter and Honey

Ingredients:

- 2 wholegrain slices

- 2 tsp. natural peanut butter

- 1 teaspoon of honey

Instructions:

1. Onto 1 slice of bread, evenly spread the peanut butter.

2. Pour honey on top of peanut butter.

3. To make a sandwich, place the second slice of bread on top.

4. If preferred, cut the sandwich in half.

5. Serve straight away.

Prep Time: 2 minutes

Cooking Time: 0 minutes

Portion Size: 1 sandwich

Nutritional Information (per sandwich):

- **Calories:** Approximately 300

- **Protein:** 10g

- **Fat:** 12g

- **Carbohydrates:** 40g

- **Fiber:** 5g

- **Sugar:** 16g

- **Sodium:** 250mg

Allergy Information: There are peanuts in this recipe. Those who are allergic to peanuts should use a different spread or skip the peanut butter altogether. Those who are allergic to any of the compounds should also omit or use an acceptable replacement.

Tips for Acid Reflux Diet Plan:

- To reduce potential reflux triggers, use pure peanut butter without additional sugars or oils.

- If you want more fiber to help with digestion and lessen the chance of acid symptoms, use whole-grain bread.

- Savor the sandwich with peanut butter and honey as a filling, well-balanced supper or snack that is easy on the stomach and could help reduce symptoms of acid reflux.

Omelette with Vegetables

Ingredients:

- 2 eggs

- 1/4 cup chopped mixed vegetables, including spinach, bell peppers, onions, and mushrooms

- 1 tablespoon of olive oil

- To taste, add salt and pepper

Instructions:

1. Beat the eggs until they are well-beaten in a bowl.

2. In a nonstick skillet, preheat the olive oil over medium heat.

3. Cook the chopped vegetables in the pan for two to three minutes, or until they are soft.

4. Over the vegetables in the pan, add the beaten eggs.

5. Let the eggs boil for two to three minutes, or until the edges begin to stiffen.

6. Lift the omelet's edges gently with a spatula, then tilt the pan so that the uncooked eggs fall to the bottom.

7. Cook for a further two to three minutes, or until the omelet is set and well-cooked.

8. To taste, add salt and pepper for flavor.

9. After folding the omelet in half, lay it on a dish.

10. If desired, serve hot with avocado slices or whole-grain toast on the side.

Prep Time: 5 minutes

Cooking Time: 5 to 7 minutes

Portion Size: 1 omelet

Nutritional Information (for Each Omelet):

- **Calories:** Approximately 200

- **Protein:** 12g

- **Fat:** 15g

- **Carbohydrates:** 5g

- **Fiber:** 2g

- **Sugar:** 2g

- **Sodium:** 300mg

Allergy Information: There is no dairy or gluten in this dish. People who are allergic to eggs or any of the vegetables should, however, omit or use an adequate replacement for those ingredients.

Tips for Acid Reflux Diet Plan:

- Pick non-acidic foods like spinach, mushrooms, and bell peppers to decrease the potential of bringing on reflux symptoms.

- Refrain from topping the omelet with cheese or creamy sauces as dairy products could increase acid reflux.

- Use less oil while cooking the omelet to cut down on fat content, since products strong in fat could worsen GERD symptoms.

- Savor the vegetable omelet as a satisfying, healthful, and moderate option for breakfast or brunch that may also help lessen the symptoms of acid reflux.

INSPIRING QUOTES TO GET YOU ALONG WITH THE DIET

- "Nourish from inside, shine from without."

- "Nourishment is the foremost effective frame of medicine."

- "Fuel your body with nourishments that fuel your soul."

- "Eat to live, don't live to eat."

- "Strong food, cheerful mien."

- "Contribute to your well-being, it pays the finest intrigue."

- "Cook with cherish, eat with gratitude."

VEGAN RECIPES

Avocado with White Bean Toast

Ingredients:

- 2 wholegrain slices

- 1/2 cup of mashed cooked white beans (cannellini or navy beans)

- 1 sliced, ripe avocado

- 1 tablespoon of juiced lemon

- Salt and pepper to taste

- Optional toppings: cherry tomatoes, sliced cucumber, red onion, micro greens

Instructions:

1. Toast the whole grain bread slices until they are golden brown.

2. Cooked white beans should be mashed until smooth in a basin with lemon juice, salt, and pepper.

3. Evenly divide the mashed white beans over the pieces of toasted bread.

4. Put a sliced avocado on top of each toast.

5. If desired, add extra salt and pepper to the avocado's seasoning.

6. Add optional garnishes such as micro greens, sliced cucumber, red onion, or cherry tomatoes.

7. Serve straight away.

Prep Time: 5 minutes

Cooking Time: 5 minutes (toast the bread)

Portion Size: 2 bread slices

Nutritional Information (per serving - 2 pieces of toast):

- **Calories:** Approximately 300

- **Protein:** 12g

- **Fat:** 15g

- **Carbohydrates:** 35g

- **Fiber:** 12g

- **Sugar:** 2g

- **Sodium:** 500mg

Allergy Information: There is no dairy or gluten in this dish. Allergies to avocado or beans, however, should stay clear of this recipe. People who are allergic to any of the optional toppings should likewise leave out or use an acceptable replacement for those ingredients.

Tips for Acid Reflux Diet Plan:

- Select whole-grain bread to receive more fiber, which helps improve digestion and minimize the symptoms of acid reflux.

- Avocado may help soothe the lining of the stomach and is an excellent source of fat. However people who suffer from acid reflux should limit how much they consume since too much fat could make symptoms worse.

- Adjust the toppings to your taste and degree of acidity tolerance. Select non-acidic vegetables to lessen the likelihood of triggering reflux.

- Savor the white bean and avocado toast as a satisfying, healthful breakfast or snack that is easy on the stomach and might even help minimize symptoms of acid reflux.

Fava Greek

Ingredients:

- 1 cup of split yellow peas

- 3 cups of water

- 1 onion, chopped finely

- 2 minced garlic cloves

- 1/4 ounces of virgin olive oil

- 1 bay leaf

- To taste, add salt and pepper

- Optional garnishes include cherry tomatoes, lemon wedges, olives, chopped fresh parsley, and extra virgin olive oil

Instructions:

1. Drain and rinse the yellow split peas under cold water.

2. The split peas, water, onion, garlic, olive oil, and bay leaf should all be mixed in a large pot.

3. Over medium-high heat, bring the mixture to a boil. Then, decrease the heat to a simmer and cover the pot slightly. Simmer for 45 to 50 minutes, or until the split peas are soft and the liquid has thickened.

4. After removing the bay leaf, season the fava to taste with salt and pepper.

5. Blend the fava in a food processor or immersion blender until it's smooth and creamy.

6. Spoon the fava onto a dish and season it with extra virgin olive oil.

7. Optional garnishes include olives, cherry tomatoes, lemon wedges, and chopped fresh parsley.

8. Heat or serve at room temperature.

Prep Time: 10 minutes

Cooking Time: 50 minutes

Portion Size: 1/2 cup

Nutritional Information (per serving - 1/2 cup):

- **Calories:** Approximately 200

- **Protein:** 10g

- **Fat:** 7g

- **Carbohydrates:** 25g

- **Fiber:** 9g

- **Sugar:** 2g

- **Sodium:** 300mg

Allergy Information: There is no dairy or gluten in this dish. However, this recipe should not be tried by anyone who is allergic to any of the components or legumes. People who are allergic to any of the optional toppings should likewise leave out or use an acceptable replacement for those ingredients.

Tips for Acid Reflux Diet Plan:

- Because yellow split peas are low in fat and non-acidic, they are a suitable protein alternative for persons who experience acid reflux.

- Since extra virgin olive oil is a heart-healthy fat that may help decrease inflammation and relax the digestive system, use it for cooking and spreading it over the fava.

- Adjust the toppings to your taste and degree of acidity tolerance. Choose non-acidic garnishes such as olives and fresh herbs to lessen the chance of acid reflux.

- Savor the Greek fava as a wonderful and healthful appetizer or side dish that is easy on the stomach and might help lessen the symptoms of acid reflux.

Palm Tapenade Hearts

Ingredients:

- 1 (14-oz) can of drained and sliced hearts of palm

- 1/4 cup of Kalamata olives, pitted

- 2 tablespoons of capers

- 2 minced garlic cloves

- 2 tsp. freshly squeezed lemon juice

- 2 tsp. extra virgin olive oil

- To taste, add salt and pepper

- Chopped fresh parsley, if wanted, as a garnish

Instructions:

1. Add the chopped hearts of palm, capers, lemon juice, olive oil, Kalamata olives, and minced garlic to a food processor.

2. Pulse the mixture until it achieves the appropriate consistency, pausing periodically to wipe down the food processor's sides.

3. To taste, add salt and pepper for flavor.

4. If desired, garnish the tapenade with finely chopped fresh parsley after transferring it to a serving dish.

5. Accompany with toasted bread, crackers, or carrot sticks.

Prep Time: 10 minutes

Cooking Time: 0 minutes

Portion Size: 2 tablespoons

Nutritional Information (per serving - 2 teaspoons):

- **Calories:** Approximately 50

- **Protein:** 1g

- **Fat:** 5g

- **Carbohydrates:** 2g

- **Fiber:** 1g

- **Sugar:** 0g

- **Sodium:** 150mg

Allergy Information: There is no dairy or gluten in this dish. But this recipe is unsuitable for individuals who are allergic to olives, capers, or hearts of palm. Those who are allergic to any of the compounds should also omit or use an acceptable replacement.

Tips for Acid Reflux Diet Plan:

- 1 low-acid, low-fat food that may be kinder on the stomach for individuals who suffer from acid reflux is hearts of palm.

- The tapenade receives flavor from the kalamata olives and capers without being excessively acidic. However, because these components might still induce symptoms in certain individuals, those who suffer acid reflux should monitor what they consume.

- Savor the heart of palm tapenade as a pleasant and healthful appetizer or snack that is easy on the stomach and might help lessen symptoms of acid reflux.

Paella

Ingredients:

- 1 tablespoon of olive oil

- 1 chopped onion

- 2 minced garlic cloves

- 1 sliced bell pepper

- 1 sliced tomato

- 1 cup of rice, Arborio

- 2 cups of vegetable or chicken stock

- 1/2 teaspoon of optional saffron threads

- 1/2 tsp. paprika

- 1/2 tsp. dried thyme

- 1/2 teaspoon of oregano, dried

- To taste, add salt and pepper

- 1 cup of cooked seafood, such as squid, mussels, or shrimp

- Optional garnish: lemon wedges and freshly chopped fresh parsley

Instructions:

1. Heat the olive oil in a wide skillet or paella pan over medium heat.

2. Simmer the chopped onion and garlic in the pan for two to three minutes, or until they are soft.

3. Cook the tomato and diced bell pepper in the pan for a further two to three minutes.

4. Add the Arborio rice, salt, pepper, dried thyme, dried oregano, paprika, and saffron threads (if using).

5. Transfer the broth, either chicken or vegetable, into the skillet and stir completely.

6. After bringing the mixture to a simmer, turn down the heat to low and put a cover on the skillet.

7. Cook, stirring regularly, for 20 to 25 minutes, or until the rice is mushy and has absorbed the liquid.

8. After the rice is done, add your favorite cooked chicken or seafood.

9. Cook for a further two to three minutes, or until the shellfish or chicken is thoroughly cooked.

10. Take off the heat and leave it a few minutes to rest.

11. Serve with lemon wedges on the side and sprinkle with freshly cut parsley.

Prep Time: 10 minutes

Cooking Time: 30 minutes

Portion Size: 1 cup

Nutritional Information (per serving - 1 cup):

- **Calories:** Approximately 300

- **Protein:** 15g

- **Fat:** 5g

- **Carbohydrates:** 45g

- **Fiber:** 3g

- **Sugar:** 2g

- **Sodium:** 500mg

Allergy Information: There is no gluten in this recipe. But this is not a recipe for anybody who is allergic to any of the components, including shellfish, chicken, or any other ingredient. Those who are allergic to any of the optional garnishes should likewise omit or use an adequate replacement for those components.

Tips for Acid Reflux Diet Plan:

- To decrease your intake of fat, choose lean proteins in your paella, such as chicken or seafood, since high-fat meals could increase GERD symptoms.

- Tailor the vegetables and meats in your paella to your preferences and degree of acid sensitivity. Lean meats and non-acidic vegetables are the greatest alternatives to lessen the possibility of refluxing.

- Savor the paella as a wonderful and substantial main dish that is easy on the stomach for individuals who suffer from acid reflux and contains protein, carbohydrates, and other necessary components.

Chili Mac in a Pot

Ingredients:

- 1 tablespoon of olive oil

- 1 chopped onion

- 2 minced garlic cloves

- 1 pound of lean ground turkey or beef

- 1 (14-oz) can of chopped tomatoes

- 1 can (15 oz.) of rinsed and drained kidney beans

- 2 cups of low-sodium vegetable or chicken broth

- 1 cup of macaroni elbow

- 2 tsp. of chili powder

- 1 teaspoon of cumin

- To taste, add salt and pepper

- Optional garnishes include sliced avocado, chopped green onions, and shredded cheese

Instructions:

1. Heat the olive oil in a wide pot or Dutch oven over medium heat.

2. To the saucepan, add the minced garlic and the chopped onion. Simmer for roughly 5 minutes, or until tender.

3. To the saucepan, add the ground turkey or beef. Cook for 5 to 7 minutes, breaking it up with a spoon, or until browned.

4. Add the kidney beans, diced tomatoes, cumin, chili powder, elbow macaroni, chicken or vegetable broth, and salt and pepper.

5. Once the mixture reaches a boil, drop the heat to a simmer and cover the pan. Simmer for ten to twelve minutes, or until the macaroni is soft and the liquid has thickened.

6. Before serving, remove the chili mac from the burner and let it rest for five minutes.

7. Serve hot with optional toppings such as sliced avocado, chopped green onions, or shredded cheese.

Prep Time: 10 minutes

Cooking Time: 25 minutes

Portion Size: 1/6 of the Recipe

Nutritional Information (per serving):

- **Calories:** Approximately 350

- **Protein:** 20g

- **Fat:** 10g

- **Carbohydrates:** 40g

- **Fiber:** 8g

- **Sugar:** 5g

- **Sodium:** 500mg

Allergy Information: If you use elbow macaroni in this meal, it may include gluten; if you use shredded cheese, it may have dairy. Those who are sensitive to dairy or gluten should not cook this meal.

Tips for Acid Reflux Diet Plan:

- To lower fat content, try for lean turkey or ground beef. High-fat diets increase GERD symptoms.

- Choose low-sodium broth to cut down on sodium since too much salt could make acid reflux symptoms worse.

- Savor the one-pot chili mac as a delicious and full meal that is low in fat, rich in protein, and high in fiber. It is also gentle on the stomach for individuals who suffer from acid reflux.

INSPIRING QUOTES TO GET YOU ALONG WITH THE DIET

- "Tune in to your body, it knows what it needs."

- "Sow seeds of wellbeing, harvest a gather of happiness."

- "Your body is your sanctuary, treat it with care."

- "Grasp the control of feeding foods."

- "You can't pour from a purge glass, feed yourself first."

- "Eat clean, feel enthusiastic."

- "Nourishment is the key to opening your body's potential."

- "In the kitchen, you're not just a cook; you're a sculptor shaping a masterpiece of well-being."

- "Every recipe is a brushstroke on the canvas of health."

- "Treat your body like a garden, take care of it carefully."

- "Cook with love for yourself and the people you love. It's the secret element that turns meals become therapeutic experiences.

- "Culinary artistry meets wellness—a recipe for a vibrant life."

DESSERT RECIPES

Loaf with Coconut & Cacao

Ingredients:

- 1/2 cup cacao powder

- 1 cup coconut flour

- 1 tsp. baking soda

- 4 eggs

- 1/4 teaspoon salt

- 1/2 cup melted coconut oil

- 1/2 cup of maple syrup or honey

- 1 cup of coconut milk

- 1 tsp. of vanilla flavor

- Shredded coconut flakes for garnish are optional

Instructions:

1. Set the oven temperature to 175°C, or 350°F. Grease and line a loaf pan with parchment paper.

2. Combine the coconut flour, baking soda, cacao powder, and salt in a large mixing bowl.

3. Beat the eggs in a separate basin. Next, incorporate vanilla extract, coconut milk, honey or maple syrup, and melted coconut oil. Blend until fully blended.

4. Add the wet components to the dry ingredients gradually while stirring to achieve smooth and complete mixing.

5. Fill the loaf pan with the batter. If desired, top with crushed coconut flakes.

6. Bake for forty-five to forty-five minutes, or until a toothpick inserted in the center comes clean.

7. Take the loaf out of the oven and allow it to cool in the pan for ten minutes before putting it on a wire rack to complete cooling.

8. Cut into pieces and present.

Prep Time: 10 minutes

Cooking Time: 40-45 minutes

Portion Size: 1 piece

Nutritional Information (per serving - 1 slice):

- **Calories:** About 200

- **Protein:** 4g

- **Fat:** 14g

- **Carbohydrates:** 17g

- **Fiber:** 6g

- **Sugar:** 10g

- **Sodium:** 200mg

Allergy Information: There are eggs and coconut in this recipe. Those who are allergic to coconut or eggs should not cook this meal.

Tips for Acid Reflux Diet Plan:

- Select natural sweeteners such as honey or maple syrup rather than manufactured sweets, since the latter may worsen symptoms of acid reflux.

- Compared to ordinary wheat flour and butter, coconut flour and oil are lower in fat and may be more appealing to persons with acid reflux.

- Savor the coconut and cacao bread as a sweet, satisfying treat that is easy on the stomach and might even help lessen symptoms of acid reflux.

Apple Cheesecake Caramelized

Ingredients:

Crust:

- 1/2 cup of crumbs from graham crackers

- 1/4 cup of sugar, granulated

- 1/2 cup melted unsalted butter

Filling for Cheesecake:

- 3 packages of softened cream cheese (8 oz. each)

- 1 cup of sugar powder

- 3 large eggs

- 1 cup of sour cream

- 1 teaspoon of vanilla essence

Apples with Caramel:

- Peeled, cored, and sliced four medium apples

- 1 teaspoon of ground cinnamon

- Cup of brown sugar

- Cup of unsalted butter

- 1 pinch of salt

Instructions:

1. Set the oven temperature to 325°F or 160°C. In a 9-inch spring form pan, oil it.

2. Place the melted butter, granulated sugar, and graham cracker crumbs in a mixing bowl. Load all of the ingredients into the prepared pan.

3. Combine the cream cheese and powdered sugar in a large mixing bowl and beat until smooth. One egg at a time, adding and beating thoroughly after each addition. Add the sour cream and vanilla essence and mix until thoroughly incorporated.

4. Cover the prepared crust in the spring form pan with the cheesecake filling.

5. In a pan placed over medium heat, melt the butter. Incorporate the diced apples, cinnamon, brown sugar, and salt. Simmer for 8 to 10 minutes, stirring now and then, or until the apples are tender and caramelized.

6. Place the caramelized apples on top of the ingredients for the cheesecake.

7. Transfer the spring form pan to a baking sheet and bake for 55 to 60 minutes in a preheated oven, or until the cheesecake is set on the exterior but still slightly jiggly on the inside.

8. Take the cheesecake out of the oven and allow it time to cool entirely. Place in the refrigerator for at least 4 hours or overnight before serving.

9. Present cold slices of apple cheesecake with caramel.

Prep Time: 30 minutes

Cooking Time: 55-60 minutes

Chilling Time: 4 hours or overnight

Portion Size: 1 slice

Nutritional Information (per serving - 1 slice):

- **Calories:** Approximately 400

- **Protein:** 6g

- **Fat:** 25g

- **Carbohydrates:** 40g

- **Fiber:** 2g

- **Sugar:** 30g

- **Sodium:** 250mg

Allergy Information: There are eggs and dairy in this dish. This recipe should not be tried by anyone who is allergic to eggs or dairy.

Tips for Acid Reflux Diet Plan:

- To lower the cheesecake's fat content, use sour cream and reduced-fat cream cheese. High-fat meals might increase acid reflux symptoms.

- Use less butter in the crust and a thinner layer of graham cracker crumbs to get a lighter crust.

- Eat the rich dessert choice of caramelized apple cheesecake in moderation, and check portion sizes to prevent reflux episodes.

Pumpkin Pie

Ingredients:

- 1 (15-oz) can of pureed pumpkin

- 1 (14-oz) can of condensed milk with added sugar

- 2 large eggs

- 1 teaspoon of ground cinnamon

- 1/2 teaspoon of ground ginger

- 1/4 teaspoon of cloves, ground

- 1/2 teaspoon of salt

- 1 pie crust, either homemade or from the store

- Optional whipped cream for serving

Instructions:

1. Set the oven temperature to 425°F (220°C).

2. Ground cinnamon, ground ginger, ground cloves, eggs, sweetened condensed milk, and salt should all be properly combined in a huge mixing bowl.

3. Evenly divide the pumpkin mixture throughout the unbaked pie crust as you pour it in.

4. Bake the pie for fifteen minutes in an oven that has been preheated.

5. Lower the oven's temperature to 350°F/175°C and bake for a further 35 to 40 minutes, or until the toothpick inserted into the center comes out clean and the filling is set.

6. Before slicing, take the pie out of the oven and allow it to cool thoroughly.

7. If wanted, top pumpkin pie slices with whipped cream.

Prep Time: 10 minutes

Cooking Time: 50–55 minutes

Portion Size: 1 pie piece

Nutritional Information (per serving - 1 slice of pie):

- **Calories:** Approximately 300

- **Protein:** 7g

- **Fat:** 10g

- **Carbohydrates:** 45g

- **Fiber:** 2g

- **Sugar:** 30g

- **Sodium:** 350mg

Allergy Information: Dairy and eggs are used in this dish. Those who are allergic to dairy or eggs should not cook this meal.

Tips for Acid Reflux Diet Plan:

- Select a low-fat pie crust, either homemade or from the store, to decrease the amount of probable acid reflux triggers.

- To expedite preparation and stay clear of unnecessary components that can worsen GERD symptoms, use pumpkin pie spice rather than the precise spices indicated in the recipe.

- As a festive dessert option, eat pumpkin pie in moderation, but check portion sizes and restrict consumption to prevent reflux flare-ups.

Pudding of Rice, Arroz with Leche

Ingredients:

- 1 cup of white rice

- 4 cups of whole milk

- 1 stick of cinnamon

- 1/2 cup sugar

- 1 tsp. of vanilla extract

- Ground cinnamon (optional) as a garnish

- Garnish with raisins, if preferred.

Instructions:

1. After washing with cold water, drain the white rice.

2. The whole milk, cinnamon stick, and rinsed rice should all be mixed in a huge saucepan.

3. After bringing the mixture to a boil over medium-high heat, drop the heat to a simmer and cook, stirring from time to time, until the rice is cooked and the liquid has thickened around 30 to 35 minutes.

4. Add the sugar and vanilla essence, stirring until fully combined.

5. Take out and discard the cinnamon stick from the rice pudding.

6. Before serving, take the rice pudding off of the burner and allow it to cool considerably.

7. If desired, top the warm or cold rice pudding with chopped almonds and ground cinnamon.

Prep Time: 5 minutes

Cooking Time: 35 minutes

Portion Size: 1/2 cup

Nutritional Information (per serving - 1/2 cup):

- **Calories:** Approximately 200

- **Protein:** 5g

- **Fat:** 4g

- **Carbohydrates:** 35g

- **Fiber:** 0g

- **Sugar:** 20g

- **Sodium:** 70mg

Allergy Information: This dish includes dairy. Individuals with sensitivities to dairy should avoid this dish.

Tips for Acid Reflux Diet Plan:

- Use whole milk for a creamier texture; however, people who experience acid reflux may pick low-fat or dairy-free milk replacements to cut down on fat and probable reflux triggers.

- Rice pudding may be a delicious dessert choice when taken in moderation. However, to reduce reflux flare-ups, control meal amounts and restrict consumption.

- Try experimenting with various spices, such as cardamom or nutmeg, to achieve flavor variations that meet your dietary restrictions and personal preferences.

Kourabiedes, Greek Butter Cookies

Ingredients:

- 1/2 cup powdered sugar, plus additional for dusting

- 1 cup melted unsalted butter

- 2 cups all-purpose flour

- 1/4 cup finely chopped blanched almonds

- 1 teaspoon vanilla extract

- 1 sprinkle of salt

Instructions:

1. Set the oven temperature to 175°C or 350°F. Use parchment paper to line a baking sheet.

2. Lightly whisk the powdered sugar and melted butter in a mixing bowl until foamy.

3. Ensure that the vanilla essence and chopped almonds are properly blended.

4. Add the salt and all-purpose flour gradually, stirring to form a smooth dough.

5. Use the dough to shape tiny crescents or balls, then lay them on the baking sheet that has been prepared.

6. Bake for 15 to 20 minutes, or until the cookies are just starting to get golden brown, in the preheated oven.

7. Take the cookies out of the oven and allow them to cool for five minutes on the baking sheet.

8. Sprinkle powdered sugar over the cookies while they're still warm.

9. Before serving, allow the cookies to cool thoroughly.

Prep Time: 15 minutes

Cooking Time: 15 to 20 minutes

Portion Size: 1 cookie

Nutritional Information (per serving - 1 cookie):

- **Calories:** Approximately 100

- **Protein:** 1g

- **Fat:** 7g

- **Carbohydrates:** 9g

- **Fiber:** 0g

- **Sugar:** 3g

- **Sodium:** 25mg

Allergy Information: There are almonds and dairy in this recipe. Those who are allergic to almonds or dairy should not cook this recipe.

Tips for Acid Reflux Diet Plan:

- Opt for unsalted butter to minimize the sodium content since too much salt could make acid reflux symptoms worse.

- Savor some Greek butter. - Cookies are a great treat when taken in moderation, but to prevent reflux flare-ups, control portion sizes, and restrict consumption. To limit sugar intake and possible reflux triggers, consider about using less powdered sugar when dusting.

Banana Oatmeal Cookies

Ingredients:

- 2 ripe bananas, mashed

- 1 cup rolled oats

- 1/4 cup unsweetened applesauce

- 1/4 teaspoon ground cinnamon

- Optional: 1/4 cup pecans or chopped walnuts

- Optional: 1/4 cup dried or raisins or dried cranberries

Instructions:

1. Preheat your oven to 350°F (175°C). Line a baking sheet with parchment paper.

2. In a mixing dish, combine the mashed bananas, rolled oats, applesauce, and ground cinnamon. Stir until completely blended.

3. If preferred, mix in the chopped nuts and raisins or dried cranberries until uniformly distributed throughout the dough.

4. Using a spoon or cookie scoop, put tablespoon-sized amounts of the dough onto the prepared baking sheet, spreading them approximately 2 inches apart.

5. Use the back of the spoon or your fingertips to gently flatten each cookie.

6. Bake in the preheated oven for 12-15 minutes, or until the cookies are golden brown around the edges.

7. Remove from the oven and allow the cookies to rest on the baking sheet for 5 minutes before moving them to a wire rack to cool entirely.

Prep Time: 10 minutes

Cooking Time: 12-15 minutes

Portion Size: Makes roughly 12 cookies

Nutritional Information (per serving, based on 1 cookie):

- **Calories:** 70 kcal

- **Carbohydrates:** 14 g

- **Fat:** 1 g

- **Protein:** 1.5 g

- **Fiber:** 1.5 g

- **Sugars:** 5.5 g

- **Sodium:** 0 mg

Allergy Information: This dish is naturally gluten-free and dairy-free. However, persons with nut allergies should skip the chopped nuts or substitute them with seeds or extra-dried fruit.

Tips for Acid Reflux Diet Plan:

- Use ripe bananas for natural sweetness and taste without additional sugar.

- Choose unsweetened applesauce to prevent unwanted added sugars.

- Opt for rolled oats instead of quick oats for increased fiber and texture.

- Customize the cookies with your favorite mix-ins, such as nuts, seeds, or dried fruit, but avoid substances that may provoke acid reflux symptoms.

- Enjoy these cookies in moderation as a pleasant and reflux-friendly dessert. Pair with a calming herbal tea or almond milk for a wonderful snack.

These Banana Oatmeal Cookies are a tasty and reflux-friendly solution for fulfilling your sweet taste without aggravation. Enjoy!

INSPIRING QUOTES TO GET YOU ALONG WITH THE DIET

- "Wellbeing is riches, contribute wisely."

- "Select nourishments that adore you back."

- "Let nourishment be your establishment for wellness."

- "Each dinner is an opportunity to nourish yourself."

- "Eat mindfully, live cheerfully."

- "Nourish your body and feed your spirit. Every bite is a step towards a healthier, happier you.

- "Culinary artistry meets wellness—a recipe for a vibrant life."

- "Your health is an investment, and every meal is an opportunity to capitalize on well-being."

- "Fuel your body with the goodness it deserves, and watch it flourish in return."

CONCLUSION

In summary, the "Complete Easy Acid Reflux Diet Plan" cookbook is more than just a list of dishes; it's a manual for regaining control over your digestive health and wellbeing. This cookbook provides a complete approach to reducing acid reflux with its exquisite meals that are precisely prepared to relax your stomach and thrill your taste buds.

Every meal, from substantial breakfasts to satisfying dinners and delightful snacks, is meticulously engineered to be easy on your stomach while carrying a punch in terms of taste and nutrition. No matter whether you're eating thick Quinoa-Stuffed Bell Pepper, a rich Caramelized Apple Cheesecake, or the sheer bliss of a Greek Butter Cookie, each bite is a step closer to alleviating your discomfort and embracing a vigorous way of life.

But this cookbook is more than merely a selection of meals; it's also a complete reference for knowing and handling the subtleties of acid reflux. You'll be prepared with all the information, meal plans, and fitness advice you need to start your road toward greater gut health and overall well-being.

Why then wait? Take charge of your health right now by beginning a culinary adventure that will not only help you conquer acid reflux but also offer you a new perspective on the value of eating excellent, healthy food. The first step to a more contented and joyful life is the "Complete Easy Acid Reflux Diet Plan" cookbook.

INSPIRING QUOTES TO GET YOU ALONG WITH THE DIET

- "Cooking with passion, nurturing with love."

- "Eat healthy, feel full of vitality."

Thanks for feeding your stomach!

As you begin on your acid reflux diet plan, may these dishes ease your stomach and enhance your health. Remember, every mouthful is a step toward improved health. Wishing you many tasty and joyful dinners!

Always balanced, always active!

SECTION III: BONUSES

5 Unique GERD Exercises

Exercises that enhance digestion, decrease stress levels, and help you maintain a healthy weight may be combined with the dietary ideas in the "Complete Easy Acid Reflux Diet Plan" cookbook to help manage your acid reflux. The following seven miraculous exercises are advised for you to simply stick to the acid reflux diet plan:

1. Strolling: One low-impact exercise that is easy to add to routine activities is strolling. On most days of the week, aim to get in at least 30 minutes of brisk walking. Walking helps with stress reduction, digestion, and keeping a healthy weight which are crucial for reducing your acid reflux.

2. Yoga: Yoga improves overall well-being by integrating physical postures, breathing methods, and meditation. Certain yoga positions, such as downward-facing dogs, sitting twists, and cat-cow, could help relieve your acid reflux symptoms and increase digestion. Additionally, stress is a common reflux trigger that may be minimized by practicing mindfulness and relaxation strategies in yoga.

3. Riding a Bike: Cycling is a cardiovascular activity that may be customized to meet varied degrees of fitness. Riding a stationary bike inside or outdoors is a low-impact workout that improves cardiovascular health and helps with weight management. Additionally, cycling has the potential to be a stress-relieving activity that lessens your probability of acid reflux symptoms.

4. Diving In Swimming: It is a wonderful full-body activity that is healthy for you and individuals of all ages and gentle on the joints. It enhances cardiovascular fitness and works for numerous muscle groups without taxing the digestive system. Swimming may also aid you with acid reflux management by encouraging calm and decreasing stress.

5. Pilates: Pilates seeks to promote flexibility, strengthen the core muscles, and improve posture. Strengthening your abdominal muscles with activities like leg circles, pelvic tilts, and abdominal curls may improve digestion and minimize the pressure on your stomach, so minimizing acid reflux. Pilates also focuses a heavy emphasis on stress-reduction tactics for breathing.

Before starting a new training regimen, you should always check with your doctor or fitness instructor, particularly if you have any underlying medical problems.

In addition, the answer to being consistent and reaping the rewards of exercise while following to this Complete Easy Acid Reflux Diet Plan is to listen to your body and pick routines that you find comfortable and delightful.

INSPIRING QUOTES TO GET YOU ALONG WITH THE DIET

- "Choose foods that meet your body's needs."

- "The ultimate act of self-care is nutrition."

- "The great form of self-esteem is eating well."

- "Appreciate the joy of healthy eating."

- "Your body deserves the best, feed it right."

- "Celebrating the richness of nutritious foods."

- "Life is too short to eat boring foods. Spice it up with some health, taste, and love."

- "Life is too short to eat boring foods. Spice it up with some health, taste, and love."

- "Food is more than just sustenance; it's a celebration of life." Make every meal a wellness celebration."

- "Eating well is a form of self-respect." "Treat your body like a temple."

- 14. "Healthy eating is an act of self-love. Choose sustenance that appeals to your heart."

14-Day Meal Plan

Day 1:

- **Breakfast:** Spinach and Tomatoes in an Egg White Scramble

- **Lunch:** Quinoa and Roasted Vegetable Bowl

- **Dinner:** Grilled Salmon with Lemon and Dill, served with a side of Brown Rice

- **Snack:** Greek Yogurt Parfait

Day 2:

- **Breakfast:** Smoothie Bowl

- **Lunch:** Quinoa-Stuffed Bell Peppers

- **Dinner:** Hearts of Palm Tapenade with Rice Cake and Almond Butter, accompanied by a side salad

- **Snack:** Blueberry Banana Smoothie

Day 3:

- **Breakfast:** Buckwheat Pancakes

- **Lunch:** Mediterranean Quinoa Salad

- **Dinner:** Vegetable Omelette served with Greek Butter Cookies (Kourabiedes)

- **Snack:** DIY Healthy Trail Mix

Day 4:

- **Breakfast:** Greek Yogurt Parfait

- **Lunch:** Sweet Potato and Chickpea Stew

- **Dinner:** Baked Chicken Breast with Herbs, served with a side of Steamed Asparagus

- **Snack:** Baked Sweet Potato Fries

Day 5:

- **Breakfast:** Oatmeal with Almond Butter and Banana

- **Lunch:** Lentil Soup with Spinach

- **Dinner:** Turkey Lettuce Wraps, accompanied by a side of Zucchini Noodles with Pesto

- **Snack:** Banana Bars

Day 6:

- **Breakfast:** Chia Seed Pudding

- **Lunch:** Grilled Chicken Salad

- **Dinner:** Paella

- **Snack:** Rice Cake with Almond Butter and Sliced Banana

Day 7:

- **Breakfast:** Quinoa Breakfast Bowl

- **Lunch:** Brown Rice Sushi Rolls

- **Dinner:** One-Pot Chili Mac

- **Snack:** Peanut Butter and Honey Sandwich

Day 8:

- **Breakfast:** Smoothie Bowl

- **Lunch:** Arroz con Leche (Rice Pudding)

- **Dinner:** Salmon and Asparagus

- **Snack:** 2-Ingredient Hummus with Vegetable Sticks

Day 9:

- **Breakfast:** Buckwheat Pancakes

- **Lunch:** Quinoa-Stuffed Bell Peppers

- **Dinner:** Caramelized Apple Cheesecake

- **Snack:** Greek Butter Cookies (Kourabiedes)

Day 10:

- **Breakfast:** Chia Seed Pudding

- **Lunch:** Mediterranean Quinoa Salad

- **Dinner:** Baked Sweet Potato with Greek Yogurt

- **Snack:** DIY Healthy Trail Mix

Day 11:

- **Breakfast:** Greek Yogurt Parfait

- **Lunch:** Vegetable Omelette

- **Dinner:** Grilled Salmon with Lemon and Dill, served with a side of Quinoa and Roasted Vegetable Bowl

- **Snack:** 2-Ingredient Hummus with Rice Cake

Day 12:

- **Breakfast:** Oatmeal with Almond Butter and Banana

- **Lunch:** Lentil Soup with Spinach

- **Dinner:** Hearts of Palm Tapenade with Greek Fava

- **Snack:** Blueberry Banana Smoothie

Day 13:

- **Breakfast:** Quinoa Breakfast Bowl

- **Lunch:** Brown Rice Sushi Rolls

- **Dinner:** Zucchini Noodles with Pesto

- **Snack:** Baked Sweet Potato Fries

Day 14:

- **Breakfast:** Smoothie Bowl

- **Lunch:** Sweet Potato and Chickpea Stew

- **Dinner:** Turkey and Vegetable Stir-Fry

- **Snack:** Banana Bars

Following the guidelines of the acid reflux diet plan, this meal plan offers you a range of tasty and nourishing alternatives. It balances fruits, vegetables, whole grains, lean proteins, and healthy fats to improve your digestive system and lessen acid reflux symptoms.

ENDING ENERGIZING SAYS FOR YOUR HEALTHY ADVENTURE:

- "Feed your body, feed your soul."

- "Food is the highest expression of self-love."

- "Good food, good mood."

- "Sow the seeds of health, reap the fruits of peace."

- "Cook with purpose, eat with gratitude."

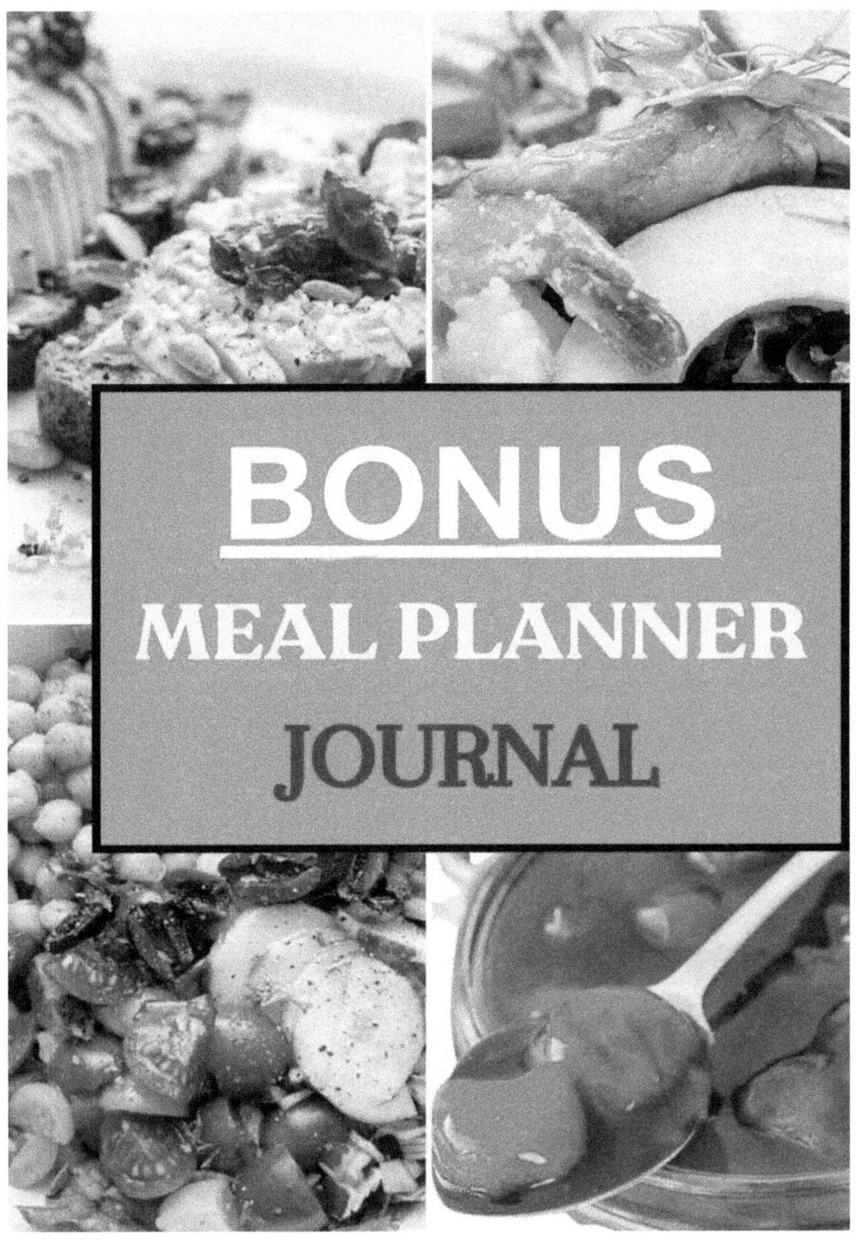
BONUS
MEAL PLANNER
JOURNAL

Weekly Meal
PLANNER JOURNAL

Week:

Date:

MONDAY
Breakfast

Lunch

Dinner

Snack

TUESDAY
Breakfast

Lunch

Dinner

Snack

WEDNESDAY
Breakfast

Lunch

Dinner

Snack

THURSDAY
Breakfast

Lunch

Dinner

Snack

FRIDAY
Breakfast

Lunch

Dinner

Snack

SATURDAY
Breakfast

Lunch

Dinner

Snack

SUNDAY
Breakfast

Lunch

Dinner

Snack

SHOPPING LIST

NOTE

Weekly Meal
PLANNER JOURNAL

Week: ______________

Date: ______________

MONDAY
Breakfast |
Lunch |
Dinner |
Snack |

TUESDAY
Breakfast |
Lunch |
Dinner |
Snack |

WEDNESDAY
Breakfast |
Lunch |
Dinner |
Snack |

THURSDAY
Breakfast |
Lunch |
Dinner |
Snack |

FRIDAY
Breakfast |
Lunch |
Dinner |
Snack |

SATURDAY
Breakfast |
Lunch |
Dinner |
Snack |

SUNDAY
Breakfast |
Lunch |
Dinner |
Snack |

SHOPPING LIST

NOTE

Weekly Meal
PLANNER JOURNAL

Week:

Date:

MONDAY
Breakfast
Lunch
Dinner
Snack

TUESDAY
Breakfast
Lunch
Dinner
Snack

WEDNESDAY
Breakfast
Lunch
Dinner
Snack

THURSDAY
Breakfast
Lunch
Dinner
Snack

FRIDAY
Breakfast
Lunch
Dinner
Snack

SATURDAY
Breakfast
Lunch
Dinner
Snack

SUNDAY
Breakfast
Lunch
Dinner
Snack

SHOPPING LIST

NOTE

Weekly Meal
PLANNER JOURNAL

Week:

Date:

MONDAY	TUESDAY	WEDNESDAY
Breakfast	Breakfast	Breakfast
Lunch	Lunch	Lunch
Dinner	Dinner	Dinner
Snack	Snack	Snack

THURSDAY	FRIDAY	SATURDAY
Breakfast	Breakfast	Breakfast
Lunch	Lunch	Lunch
Dinner	Dinner	Dinner
Snack	Snack	Snack

SUNDAY	SHOPPING LIST	NOTE
Breakfast		
Lunch		
Dinner		
Snack		

Weekly Meal
PLANNER JOURNAL

Week:

Date:

MONDAY
Breakfast

Lunch

Dinner

Snack

TUESDAY
Breakfast

Lunch

Dinner

Snack

WEDNESDAY
Breakfast

Lunch

Dinner

Snack

THURSDAY
Breakfast

Lunch

Dinner

Snack

FRIDAY
Breakfast

Lunch

Dinner

Snack

SATURDAY
Breakfast

Lunch

Dinner

Snack

SUNDAY
Breakfast

Lunch

Dinner

Snack

SHOPPING LIST

NOTE

Weekly Meal
PLANNER JOURNAL

Week:

Date:

MONDAY

Breakfast

Lunch

Dinner

Snack

TUESDAY

Breakfast

Lunch

Dinner

Snack

WEDNESDAY

Breakfast

Lunch

Dinner

Snack

THURSDAY

Breakfast

Lunch

Dinner

Snack

FRIDAY

Breakfast

Lunch

Dinner

Snack

SATURDAY

Breakfast

Lunch

Dinner

Snack

SUNDAY

Breakfast

Lunch

Dinner

Snack

SHOPPING LIST

NOTE

Weekly Meal
PLANNER JOURNAL

Week:

Date:

MONDAY

Breakfast

Lunch

Dinner

Snack

TUESDAY

Breakfast

Lunch

Dinner

Snack

WEDNESDAY

Breakfast

Lunch

Dinner

Snack

THURSDAY

Breakfast

Lunch

Dinner

Snack

FRIDAY

Breakfast

Lunch

Dinner

Snack

SATURDAY

Breakfast

Lunch

Dinner

Snack

SUNDAY

Breakfast

Lunch

Dinner

Snack

SHOPPING LIST

NOTE

Weekly Meal
PLANNER JOURNAL

Week: ___________________

Date: ___________________

MONDAY
Breakfast |
Lunch |
Dinner |
Snack |

TUESDAY
Breakfast |
Lunch |
Dinner |
Snack |

WEDNESDAY
Breakfast |
Lunch |
Dinner |
Snack |

THURSDAY
Breakfast |
Lunch |
Dinner |
Snack |

FRIDAY
Breakfast |
Lunch |
Dinner |
Snack |

SATURDAY
Breakfast |
Lunch |
Dinner |
Snack |

SUNDAY
Breakfast |
Lunch |
Dinner |
Snack |

SHOPPING LIST

NOTE

Weekly Meal
PLANNER JOURNAL

Week:

Date:

MONDAY

Breakfast

Lunch

Dinner

Snack

TUESDAY

Breakfast

Lunch

Dinner

Snack

WEDNESDAY

Breakfast

Lunch

Dinner

Snack

THURSDAY

Breakfast

Lunch

Dinner

Snack

FRIDAY

Breakfast

Lunch

Dinner

Snack

SATURDAY

Breakfast

Lunch

Dinner

Snack

SUNDAY

Breakfast

Lunch

Dinner

Snack

SHOPPING LIST

NOTE

Weekly Meal
PLANNER JOURNAL

Week: ______

Date: ______

MONDAY
Breakfast

Lunch

Dinner

Snack

TUESDAY
Breakfast

Lunch

Dinner

Snack

WEDNESDAY
Breakfast

Lunch

Dinner

Snack

THURSDAY
Breakfast

Lunch

Dinner

Snack

FRIDAY
Breakfast

Lunch

Dinner

Snack

SATURDAY
Breakfast

Lunch

Dinner

Snack

SUNDAY
Breakfast

Lunch

Dinner

Snack

SHOPPING LIST

NOTE